Implications of the Pandemic for Terrorist Interest in Biological Weapons

Islamic State and al-Qaeda Pandemic Case Studies

JOHN V. PARACHINI, ROHAN GUNARATNA

Prepared for the U.S. Department of Defense
Approved for public release; distribution unlimited

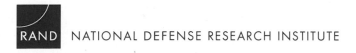

NATIONAL DEFENSE RESEARCH INSTITUTE

For more information on this publication, visit **www.rand.org/t/RRA612-1**.

About RAND

The RAND Corporation is a research organization that develops solutions to public policy challenges to help make communities throughout the world safer and more secure, healthier and more prosperous. RAND is nonprofit, nonpartisan, and committed to the public interest. To learn more about RAND, visit www.rand.org.

Research Integrity

Our mission to help improve policy and decisionmaking through research and analysis is enabled through our core values of quality and objectivity and our unwavering commitment to the highest level of integrity and ethical behavior. To help ensure our research and analysis are rigorous, objective, and nonpartisan, we subject our research publications to a robust and exacting quality-assurance process; avoid both the appearance and reality of financial and other conflicts of interest through staff training, project screening, and a policy of mandatory disclosure; and pursue transparency in our research engagements through our commitment to the open publication of our research findings and recommendations, disclosure of the source of funding of published research, and policies to ensure intellectual independence. For more information, visit www.rand.org/about/principles.

RAND's publications do not necessarily reflect the opinions of its research clients and sponsors.

About This Report

The devastating consequences of the COVID-19 pandemic and the flawed response to it in many countries exposed vulnerabilities in biopreparedness. Some policymakers and scholars wondered at the outset of the pandemic whether terrorists might be stimulated to turn to biological weapons as they saw the consequences of the outbreak and the weaknesses that major countries had contending with it. In this report, we examine Islamic State (IS) and al-Qaeda narratives associated with the pandemic for indications of whether those groups might be interested in biological weapons in the wake of the global outbreak.

An examination of past IS and al-Qaeda experiences with exotic and unconventional weaponry provides historical context for assessing the prospect of these groups using biological materials as weapons. After reviewing the historical record, we examine other exogenous factors that might further add to these groups' interest in this form of weaponry. We conclude by outlining measures that national governments and international bodies can take that have relevance to both public health and military challenges—steps designed to better prevent and prepare for future pandemics while providing capabilities to contend with a bioterrorist attack.

The research reported here was completed in September 2021 and underwent security review with the sponsor and the Defense Office of Prepublication and Security Review before public release.

RAND National Security Research Division

This research was sponsored by the U.S. Department of Defense and conducted within the International Security and Defense Policy Center of the RAND National Security Research Division (NSRD), which operates the National Defense Research Institute (NDRI), a federally funded research and development center sponsored by the Office of the Secretary of Defense, the Joint Staff, the Unified Combatant Commands, the Navy, the Marine Corps, the defense agencies, and the defense intelligence enterprise.

For more information on the RAND International Security and Defense Policy Center, see www.rand.org/nsrd/isdp or contact the director (contact information is provided on the webpage).

Acknowledgments

The authors wish to thank Laura Baldwin for supporting this project at the early stages of the COVID-19 pandemic when there were many different projects worthy of exploration. A good researcher leader, she was willing to support examination of a murky topic with potentially important implications. We also want to thank Barbara Bicksler for her review and guidance on how to shape the written product. Kofi Amora provided much-appreciated assistance with the document. Finally, we thank Alison Hottes and Milton Leitenberg for their thoughtful peer reviews of the document. We also want to thank Arwen Bicknell for her thorough edit and good suggestions on how to improve our document.

Summary

At the start of the coronavirus disease 2019 (COVID-19) pandemic caused by the severe acute respiratory syndrome coronavirus 2 (SARS-CoV-2), media statements from the Islamic State (IS) and al-Qaeda highlighted the devastating impact that the disease had on the economies of major countries around the globe. These statements put this unprecedented global event in context for followers and gave them instructions on how to survive. These groups' interpretation of events was that the pandemic was a divine means of affirming their worldview, but this initial reaction did not translate into a determined pursuit of biological agents as a means of violence, as some policymakers and analysts had feared might happen.

Over the course of the past 25 years, various violent Islamist terrorists have expressed interest in unconventional weapons. The publicly available evidence that the IS sought biological weapons is very thin and might never be known with a high degree of confidence. However, the group did use chlorine, an industrial chemical, as a weapon; the IS also produced and used some sulfur mustard agent. This use of chemical agents as a weapon is the first significant use by a nonstate actor since the Aum Shinrikyo, a Japanese cult group, released liquid sarin nerve agent on the Tokyo subway in 1995. Although the IS's development and use of sulfur agent is technologically easier to achieve than biological weapons, it serves in this study as a proxy for assessing the likelihood of members seeking to develop, produce, weaponize, and use biological materials as weapons. Al-Qaeda sought to add biological weapons to its terrorist arsenal but ultimately abandoned the effort.

Expressions of interest in biological and chemical weapons by militant Islamist groups have not translated into successful efforts. Rather, these groups have taken a portfolio management approach to violent means. In the past, they have considered many things, expressed interest in them, and ultimately pursued and employed means that were readily available, easy to wield, and that could quickly produce violent outcomes. This stands in marked contrast to the Aum leadership's obsession with biological and chemical agents. The contrast provides cold comfort that, even in the wake of a pandemic, leaders and members of the IS and al-Qaeda will pursue their deadly objectives by means other than biological weapons.

The panoply of challenges that national governments confronted as they contended with effects of the COVID-19 pandemic provide an opportunity to assess which measures might be most effective in preventing and responding to future outbreaks. Many of these measures might have a dual-use benefit in that they will not only better position governments to respond to future infectious disease outbreaks but also help to detect, prevent, deter, and respond to a terrorist use of a biological weapon. A few measures that are comparatively easy to implement are the following:

- reviewing and enhancing the processes and regulations on the increasing number of high-containment laboratories around the globe
- fostering greater collaboration between the animal and human health sectors
- ensuring the right balance of focus on near-term conventional threats and less-likely, low-probability threats with high consequences
- reinforcing international norms prohibiting development, production, and use of chemical and biological materials as weapons
- changing the conceptual approach to gauging the threat.

Too often, past policy has focused inordinately on preparing for terrorist uses of biological weapons that are more feared but are less likely, while not enough attention and resources have been dedicated to contending with a natural outbreak. Bearing in mind the results of the COVID-19 pandemic, policymakers have an opportunity to rebalance attention and focus on naturally occurring outbreaks that are likely to occur in the future.

Contents

CHAPTER ONE

Introduction

In his April 9, 2020, remarks on the global coronavirus disease 2019 (COVID-19) pandemic, United Nations Security General António Guterres opined that the "the weakness and lack of preparedness exposed by this pandemic provide a window onto how a bioterrorist attack might unfold—and may increase the risks. Nonstate groups could gain access to virulent strains that could pose similar devastation to societies around the globe."[1] As many countries have been hit by two and three waves of the disease and as the results of mass vaccinations evolve, the proposition that the pandemic has stimulated (or will stimulate) increased terrorist interest in using biological material as a weapon needs to be examined.

Far too often, the reaction to a threatening phenomenon is to associate it with what has been feared in the past. It is natural to consider past experience as an analytic anchor yet very hard to imagine the future consequences of something that has never happened before. In the case of terrorist use of unconventional weapons involving chemical and biological materials, however, the responses to the COVID-19 pandemic caused by the severe acute respiratory syndrome coronavirus 2 (SARS-CoV-2) make clear that societies tend to overprepare to counter intentional use of these weapons and do not adequately prepare for more-likely dangers, such as a natural outbreak of disease.

The risk posed by adherents of the Islamic State (IS), al-Qaeda, or any other nonstate actor is a combination of motivation, capability, opportunity to obtain the capabilities, vulnerabilities that might be exploited, and possi-

---

[1] United Nations Secretary-General, "Secretary-General's Remarks to the Security Council on the COVID-19 Pandemic," webpage, April 9, 2020.

ble consequences.[2] These groups have expressed desires to inflict mass casualties as retribution, but they have not been able to muster the capabilities to exploit some vulnerabilities revealed during the COVID-19 pandemic. If these groups could develop biological agent capabilities, they might be able to exploit vulnerabilities in governments' ability to disrupt, deter, or respond to attacks that use a virus that is transmissible in ways similar to COVID-19; this could lead to serious consequences. However, not all biological agents are transmissible like SARS-CoV-2 is. Fortunately, nonstate actors have not been able to mount a mass casualty attack with biological agents. The question is whether they might try to do so after witnessing the difficulties that governments have had contending with the COVID-19 pandemic.

Some former U.S. officials and counterterrorism analysts have expressed concern that the COVID-19 pandemic would stimulate new interest on the part of such nonstate actors as the IS and al-Qaeda to take an interest in biological materials as weapons. Former Assistant to the U.S. Secretary of Defense for Chemical and Biological Weapons Andrew Weber observed that "[o]ur fumbling of the response [to COVID-19] just advertises to the world how vulnerable we are to biological attacks. So countries that have been thinking about pursuing biological weapons or that have small programs might see the opportunity, and I would include non-state actors and terrorist groups in that."[3] Similarly, another former senior U.S. counterterrorism official argued that "[t]he imagination of apocalyptic terrorists and

---

[2] In an excellent article, Koblentz and Kiesel provide a similar framework for assessing the risk of terrorists acquiring and using biological weapons (Gregory D. Koblentz and Stevie Kiesel, "The COVID-19 Pandemic: Catalyst or Complication for Bioterrorism?" *Studies in Conflict & Terrorism*, July 14, 2021). The article covers many different terrorist groups and their pursuit of biological weapons—for example, it contains material on "far-right extremists"—but many of the arguments that the authors articulate to assess the threat of bioterrorism are consistent with ones in this report. We focus on the two violent Islamic extremist groups that have posed such a significant threat that the U.S. military and other allied country militaries have been called on to suppress them.

[3] Elizabeth Ralph, "How Covid-19 Could Give Kim Jong Un a Doomsday Weapon," *Politico*, July 28, 2020.

extremists will be reignited with the COVID-19 crisis, witnessing the mass number of deaths along with wholesale economic and social dislocation."[4]

The fear of COVID-19 increasing nonstate actor interest in using biological agents as weapons stems from both fear of the disease and the generally poor government response to the outbreak. The few incidents in which individuals who were sickened with the virus attempted to spread it to others proved ineffective.[5] An individual sickened with COVID-19 acting as a disease vector amid the pandemic might add to the outbreak, but the outbreak itself has already produced a global calamity that nations around the world are struggling to address. The spread of the disease exposed vulnerabilities of states, including some with sophisticated health care systems, and a governmental lack of preparedness to respond. All this poses two questions:

- What if the IS or al-Qaeda obtained and spread a highly contagious virus in a community or country that they sought to punish?
- Will they now seek to obtain infectious viruses to achieve these same deadly results?

The historical record of nonstate actors seeking and using poison and disease as weapons is very rare. Fortunately, in the few instances when these efforts have occurred, they were largely unsuccessful. But during a global pandemic that is a once-in-a-century phenomenon, might this moment be different? Prior to the September 11, 2001, terrorist attacks (9/11), al-Qaeda explored using chemical and biological agents as weapons. Fifteen years after 9/11, the IS used crude chemical weapons in Iraq and Syria before it was largely defeated and driven underground. Adherents of both groups have perpetrated ghastly attacks on innocent people and expressed desires to do so with results that are even more devastating. They have, thus far,

---

[4] Juan Zarate quoted in Paul Cruickshank and Don Rassler, "A View from the CT Foxhole: A Virtual Roundtable on COVID-19 and Counterterrorism with Audrey Cronin, Lieutenant General (Ret) Michael Nagata, Magnus Ranstorp, Ali Soufran, and Juan Zarate," *CTC Sentinel*, Vol. 13, No. 6, June 2020, p. 8.

[5] "Tunisia Arrests 2 for Trying to Infect Police with Virus," Agence France Presse, April 16, 2020.

chosen other means to achieve mass and indiscriminate casualties, but will this change in the wake of the pandemic?

Several nonstate actors have expressed interest in, sought to acquire, or used biological materials as weapons. In this report, we examine the interest that the IS and al-Qaeda have expressed in three types of biological agents—viruses, bacteria, and toxins. What makes biological agents such dreaded weapons is that they can result in agonizing deaths and, in some forms, can be spread without being visible. Their natural origins also make it difficult to discern whether their spread is the result of pernicious, intentional use or a natural outbreak. What complicates the detection of an intentional attack is that many of the initial symptoms resemble a variety of naturally occurring health problems. Once distributed, viruses can be spread person to person in ways that might be difficult to recognize. Although many viruses can be countered with vaccines and most bacteria can be addressed with antibiotics, not all toxins can be countered with antidotes. If they are effectively developed, produced, and disseminated, these biological agents also have the potential to kill on a mass scale.

So far, only the Rajneeshees, an obscure cult, have been even partially successful. In 1984, this group contaminated salad bars in The Dalles, Oreg., with the bacteria salmonella prior to a local election as a means of reducing local voting tallies so that their candidates might win the election.[6] This effort sickened 751 people; fortunately, however, no one died in this attack (and it failed to sway the election). However, the attack was mistaken as a natural contamination and not discovered as an intentional attack for more than a year.[7]

Policymakers and analysts have expressed concern about possible nonstate actor acquisition and use of biological weapon materials since the Soviet Union's breakup, which prompted a fear that Soviet biological weapon pro-

---

[6] Thomas J. Török, Robert V. Tauxe, Robert P. Wise, John R. Livengood, Robert Sokolow, Steven Mauvais, Kristin A. Birkness, Michael R. Skeels, John M. Horan, and Laurence R. Foster, "A Large Community Outbreak of Salmonellosis Caused by Intentional Contamination of Restaurant Salad Bars," *Journal of the American Medical Association*, Vol. 278, No. 5, August 6, 1997.

[7] W. Seth Carus, "The Rajneeshees (1984)," in Jonathan B. Tucker, ed., *Toxic Terror: Assessing Terrorist Use of Chemical and Biological Weapons*, Cambridge, Mass.: MIT Press, 2000.

gram materials might go to the highest bidder. These fears increased after a 1995 attack on the Tokyo subway with the liquid nerve agent sarin by Aum Shinrikyo, a Japanese cult. Following this attack, investigators discovered that Aum unsuccessfully experimented with an attenuated Sterne strain of anthrax.[8] Otherwise, the only known use of unconventional weapon material by a nonstate actor occurred in a series of chlorine and low-grade sulfur mustard agent attacks by the IS in Syria and Iraq.[9] Again, the lingering concern is that the COVID-19 pandemic exposed weaknesses and vulnerabilities in a government's ability to understand the origins and implications of disease outbreaks.

The last comparable event to the COVID-19 pandemic was the 1918 influenza pandemic that swept the globe killing "an estimated 50 million people worldwide, including an estimated 675,000 people in the United States."[10] At first, symptoms were so mild that the disease was misdiagnosed; then, it surged without warning in an intensely virulent and lethal fashion.[11] There

---

[8]   Anthony T. Tu, "Aum Shinrikyo's Chemical and Biological Weapons: More Than Sarin," *Forensic Science Review*, Vol. 26, No. 115, 2014, p. 120. For more on Aum, see Milton Leitenberg, *Assessing the Biological Weapons and Bioterrorist Threat*, Carlyle, Pa.: Strategic Studies Institute, U.S. Army War College, 2005, p. 30; John Parachini and Katsu Furakawa, "Japan and Aum Shinrikyo," in Robert J. Art and Louise Richardson, eds., *Democracy and Counterterrorism: Lessons from the Past*, Washington, D.C.: U.S. Institute of Peace, January 2007; Richard Danzig, Marc Sageman, Terrance Leigh, Lloyd Hough, Hidemi Yuki, Rui Kotani and Zachary M. Hosford, *Aum Shinrikyo: Insights into How Terrorists Develop Biological and Chemical Weapons*, 2nd ed., Washington, D.C.: Center for New American Security, December 2012, p. 25; John Parachini, "Aum Shinrikyo," in Brian A. Jackson, John C. Baker, Peter Chalk, Kim Cragin, John Parachini, and Horacio R. Trujillo, *Aptitude for Destruction*, Vol. 2, *Case Studies of Learning in Terrorist Organizations*, Santa Monica, Calif.: RAND Corporation, MG-332-NIJ, 2005.

[9]   Joby Warrick, *Red Line: The Unraveling of Syria and America's Race to Destroy the Most Dangerous Arsenal in the World*, New York: Doubleday, 2021, p. 235.

[10]   Douglas Jordan, Terrence Tumpey, and Barbara Jester, *The Deadliest Flu: The Complete Story of the Discovery and Reconstruction of the 1918 Pandemic Virus*, Washington, D.C.: Centers for Disease Control and Prevention, National Center for Immunization and Respiratory Diseases, December 17, 2019.

[11]   John M. Barry, "1918 Revisited: Lessons and Suggestions for Further Inquiry," in Stacey L. Knobler, Alison Mack, Adel Mahmoud, and Stanley M. Lemon, eds., *The Threat of Pandemic Influenza: Are We Ready? Workshop Summary*, Washington, D.C.: National Academies Press, 2005.

were multiple warnings of the danger of a pandemic before the onset of the COVID-19 outbreak, but when there are many potential threats on the horizon, it is difficult to appreciate the probability of one that has not been profoundly experienced by the current generation. Every four or five years, the National Intelligence Council produces a document to inform senior U.S. government decision leaders of future global trends. Except for the first one produced in 1997, every one of these documents has warned of a possible pandemic.[12] Other noted U.S. leaders issued statements warning about the likelihood of a global pandemic.[13]

In contrast to multiple alerts about the prospect of an infectious disease pandemic, the 9/11 attacks seemingly came without warning. In 2001, al-Qaeda used an unprecedented method of inflicting mass casualties by hijacking passenger airliners laden with jet fuel and crashing them into the World Trade Center towers in New York and the Pentagon in Arlington, Va. (with a third attempt thwarted and the plane going down in Shanksville, Pa.). Although U.S. officials were aware of signs of interest in attacking the towers, the method that al-Qaeda used was not anticipated. Several other attacks— such as those that involved using conventional explosives, coordinating attacks with firearms, and driving vehicles into crowds of people—showed that the IS, al-Qaeda, and those inspired by such groups could inflict high-profile mass casualties without resorting to exotic materials, such as chemical or biological agents. The seemingly surprising nature of the 9/11 attacks shocked Americans and produced fear that was fundamentally different from fears related to the COVID-19 pandemic. Al-Qaeda produced an extraordinary level of fear with an unprecedented use of conventional means. In the years following 9/11, terrorist groups continued to harbor interests in exotic weapons but staged numerous gruesome attacks with conventional means.

The IS broke with this historical pattern by using sulfur mustard and chlorine as many as 71 times from 2015 to 2017, on the battlefield and in civilian

---

[12] For example, see National Intelligence Council, *Mapping the Global Future: Report of the National Intelligence Council's 2020 Project*, Washington, D.C., NIC 2004-13, December 2004.

[13] ArLuther Lee, "Obama Warned of Pandemic Threat in 2014 but Republicans Blocked Funding," *Atlanta Journal-Constitution*, April 15, 2020; Tyler Sonnemaker, "Bill Gates Said He Warned Trump About the Dangers of a Pandemic in December 2016 Before He Took Office," *Business Insider*, May 11, 2020.

areas in Syria and Iraq.[14] The battlefield use was generally ineffective, and most of the casualties were civilians.[15] Nevertheless, a new threshold was crossed. In 2016, Director of National Intelligence James Clapper testified that the IS "used toxic chemicals in Iraq and Syria, including the blister agent sulfur mustard—the first time an extremist group has produced and used a chemical warfare agent in an attack since Aum Shinrikyo used Sarin in Japan in 1995."[16] Aside from a few thwarted crude plots to produce ricin, the IS, al-Qaeda, and other aligned groups or inspired individuals have not made biological materials a weapon of choice. IS use of crude chemical agents in Syria and Iraq raised concern about the possibility of a new trend.

IS use of chemicals in the 2015–2017 period did not match the levels that officials anticipated decades earlier. In the 1990s and early 2000s, considerable U.S. government attention and resources were dedicated to preparing for terrorist attacks with biological agents, especially involving known biological warfare agents, such as anthrax and smallpox.[17] However, the initial

---

[14] Jack Moore, "ISIS' Chemical Weapons Capability Collapses in Syria After Battlefield Losses," *Newsweek*, August 13, 2017. There are multiple sources providing different numbers of IS chemical attacks ranging from a dozen to our noted 71.

[15] Oddly, the IS did not use chemical weapons at times when it might have been expected to do so—not even when it was losing the capital of its "Caliphate," the Iraqi city of Mosul, to Iraqi forces in spring 2017.

[16] James R. Clapper, "Remarks as Delivered by The Honorable James R. Clapper, Director of National Intelligence, Senate Select Committee on Intelligence—IC's Worldwide Threat Assessment, Opening Statement," Washington, D.C., February 9, 2016, p. 3.

[17] In February 1999, the newly established Johns Hopkins Center for Civilian Biodefense Studies hosted the first National Symposium on Medical and Public Health Response to Bioterrorism. The presentations from the proceedings were published in *Emerging Infectious Diseases*, a peer-reviewed journal published by the National Center for Infectious Diseases. A presentation by U.S. Secretary of Health and Humans Services Donna E. Shalala explained how that U.S. government officials realized that a bioterrorist attack could really happen, which is why they spent "$158 million this fiscal year to prepare for bioterrorism and why the president has proposed increasing that investment by an additional $72 million in his Fiscal Year 2000 budget." Donna E. Shalala, "Bioterrorism: How Prepared Are We?" *Emerging Infectious Diseases*, Vol. 5, No. 4, July–August 1999. Also see Aidan McCarty, "Changes in U.S. Biosecurity Following the 2001 Anthrax Attacks," *Journal of Bioterrorism & Biodefense*, Vol. 9, No. 2, June 25, 2018; John Dudley Miller, "Postal Anthrax Aftermath: Has Biodefense Spending Made Us Safer?" *Scientific American*, November 1, 2008; and Susan Wright, "Taking Biodefense Too Far," *Bulletin of the Atomic Scientists*, November/December 2004.

concern focused on possible terrorist acquisition and use of unconventional weapons to cause mass casualties, which diverted attention, imagination, funding, and planning away from conventional means of attack and from natural disease outbreaks that were more likely to occur. The danger of focusing too much attention on whether the IS and al-Qaeda seek to use biological materials to inflict mass casualties is that it, too, diverts attention and resources to less-likely means of attack and away from emergencies that are more likely to arise.

The COVID-19 pandemic exposed vulnerabilities of developed countries with extensive public health care infrastructure. Fear that terrorists might exploit these vulnerabilities has thus far proven unfounded, but addressing these vulnerabilities will be important in the months and years to come. The flawed response to COVID-19 in the United States stems from a failure of political leadership, but the nation's capacity to address a pandemic was also hampered by an inordinate focus and preparation on an unlikely biological attack (albeit with potentially high consequences) by a nation-state or non-state actor. Several accounts of the mistakes and deliberate obfuscations of the seriousness of COVID-19 on the part of U.S. political leadership—particularly by President Donald J. Trump—provide detailed timelines of steps not taken, mistakes made, and attempts to shift blame for the galloping pace of the pandemic in spring 2020. These accounts make clear that the pandemic could have been less severe if the U.S. government response had been different.[18]

Leadership decisions were the biggest missteps in responding to COVID-19 in the United States, but the country's ability to respond effectively was also limited by a history of government decisions that invested scarce resources for response to a bioterrorist attack rather than to a natural outbreak of infectious disease. Chris Hamby and Sheryl Gay Stolberg revealed in a groundbreaking *New York Times* investigation how several policymakers overemphasized U.S. preparations for bioterrorist attacks with known warfare agents and did not adequately prepare the nation for

---

[18] Michael Lewis, *The Premonition: A Pandemic Story*, New York: W.W. Norton & Company, 2021. Lawrence Wright, "The Plague Year: The Mistakes and the Struggles Behind America's Coronavirus Tragedy," *The New Yorker*, December 28, 2020. Also see David Leonhardt, "A Complete List of Trump's Attempts to Play Down Coronavirus: He Could Have Taken Action. He Didn't," *New York Times*, March 15, 2020.

natural outbreaks of infectious disease. The reporters quoted former CDC director Dr. Thomas Frieden, who said that the "risk of a serious terrorist attack with anthrax is real, but that doesn't mean you buy unlimited quantities of vaccines. . . . There is only so much money, and so if you buy more of one thing, you have less to buy of another" referring to capabilities to address an unexpected outbreak like COVID-19.[19]

Similarly, Dr. Robert Kadlec, the official responsible for making relevant resource allocations in the years immediately prior to the COVID-19 pandemic, said, "If I could spend less on anthrax replenishment, I could buy more N95s [masks]. I could buy more ventilators. I could buy more of other things that quite frankly I didn't have the money to buy."[20] Kadlec's admission is ironic because he has consistently warned about the likelihood of a bioterrorist attack and the need to prepare to counter it. In congressional testimony in 2014, he said that "[t]he risk of bioattacks in the United States is an uncertain yet imminent reality." In the same hearing, he testified that "[c]onflating deliberate and natural disease threats somehow implies that by addressing the more common Mother Nature problem, the solution will be sufficient to address the deliberate biological threat. It is not."[21] Regardless of whether the United States was prepared for an intentional bioterrorist attack, we now know that it was not prepared to effectively manage "natural disease threats."

New York Times analysis found that "from 2010 through 2018, the anthrax vaccine consumed more than 40 percent of the stockpile's budget, which averaged $560 million during those years." Some experts argued more than a decade ago that an anthrax attack posed a low enough risk to civilian society that it could be adequately addressed by other means than vaccine stockpile. In 2007, Dr. Anthony S. Fauci stated in congressional tes-

---

[19] Chris Hamby and Sheryl Gay Stolberg, "Preparing for Bioterror, Neglecting Virus Threat," *New York Times*, March 7, 2021, p. 1.

[20] Hamby and Stolberg, 2021, p. 1.

[21] Robert Kadlec, testimony of Dr. Robert Kadlec before the Subcommittee on Emergency Preparedness, Response, and Communications, Committee on Homeland Security, House of Representatives, 113th Congress, 2nd session, Washington, D.C., February 11, 2014.

timony that, rather than stocking up on anthrax vaccine supplies, "The best approach toward anthrax is antimicrobial therapy."[22]

U.S. emphasis on maintaining a robust stockpile of anthrax vaccine for years—rather than pursuing a more balanced strategy that allocated more attention and resources to the more likely event of a naturally occurring outbreak—is illustrative of how fear of a low-probability terrorist attack skewed resources away from a health security risk that many had warned about for years.[23] Biotechnology companies capitalized on the fear of policymakers by arguing that the national stockpile of anthrax vaccine required regular replenishment. In post-9/11 America, congressional and executive branch policymakers viewed no downside to hedging against the prospect of the possible, albeit unlikely, event of terrorist use of a biological warfare agent. The consequence was that government funding went to meet capabilities narrowly suited to counter a bioterrorist attack with a particular agent rather than to stockpiling equipment needed for a natural outbreak and planning how to contend with such an event.

Preparations for a naturally occurring infectious disease, such as COVID-19, proved woefully inadequate. Some of the widely recognized preparedness deficiencies are insufficient amounts of testing kits, personal protective equipment, and tracing procedures; lack of federal, state, and local government preparation for how to coordinate a response to a natural outbreak; and lack of medical equipment to support individuals who contract an infectious respiratory disease. As Fauci noted, the development of antimicrobial therapies might prove more useful than the development of vaccines for known biological agents. Basic research on broad-spectrum antimicrobial therapies can lead to the development of means to address illness stemming from bacteria, viruses, fungi, and parasitic agents. This approach is more versatile and covers more possibilities than the development of vaccines for known agents. The COVID-19 pandemic illustrated the difficulty of developing just the right vaccine for a new and unknown virus. After the disease is studied, an appropriate vaccine can be developed. The rapid development of vaccines to counter COVID-19 demonstrates the

---

[22] Hamby and Stolberg, 2021.

[23] Hamby and Stolberg, 2021.

possibility of developing a countermeasure to a virus once its properties are understood.[24]

The IS and al-Qaeda reacted to the onset of the global pandemic and used it in their narratives. Since the initial outbreak in early 2020, however, media organs of both organizations have moved on to new lines. Will they return to this topic and amplify their narrative by weaving in the pandemic's effects? Will ideas about the use of biological material loom larger in the minds of their leaders or followers during a future wave of the pandemic?

Examining the narratives arising from these two groups' reactions to COVID-19 provides insight regarding whether the pandemic increases the likelihood that they will seek and use biological materials. As the initial concern at the outset of the pandemic is put in perspective, it might be possible to better discern whether the bioterrorism threat has changed. The historical record suggests that nonstate actor interest waxes and wanes regarding poison and disease as weapons. In contrast, the use of conventional explosives or unconventional uses of such readily available means as trucks, airplanes, aerial drones, and small arms has become more common in many incidents of mass casualties that continue to inflict death and destruction around the globe.

Organization of This Report

This report of our assessment of whether the COVID-19 pandemic has stimulated IS and al-Qaeda interest in biological weapons is organized into four sections. We discuss general categories of biological agents that have been used as biological weapons. These agents are viruses, bacteria, and toxins.[25] Narrowing the focus to biological agents still includes biological materials that have

---

[24] Karin Bok, Sandra Sitar, Barney S. Graham, and John R. Mascola, "Accelerated COVID-19 Vaccine Development: Milestones, Lessons, and Prospects," *Immunity*, August 10, 2021. Also see Nicole Lurie, Melanie Saville, Richard Hatchett, and Jane Halton, "Developing Covid-19 Vaccines at Pandemic Speed," *New England Journal of Medicine*, May 21, 2000.

[25] Toxins are proteins and deemed warfare agents by both the Biological Weapons Convention and the Chemical Weapons Convention. See Organisation for the Prohibition of Chemical Weapons (OPCW), Scientific Advisory Board, "Ricin Fact Sheet," Twenty-First Session, SAB-21/WP.5, February 28, 2014.

the properties of viruses, bacteria, and toxins but might not be widely recognized as biological weapons yet are employed by attackers as weapons. In some places, we refer to *biological agent material* to distinguish the toxic or infectious material from the *weapon*, which is a system that results from weaponization of the material. An expansive definition of biological agents is important because some novel biological agents might be employed in the future that are not among those commonly discussed today. The IS and al-Qaeda both frequently conflate so-called weapons of mass destruction (WMD) in their narratives to feature chemical, biological, radiological, and nuclear weapons without clearly making a distinction among them. In many cases, they simply mean any weapon that can produce mass and indiscriminate casualties. In Chapter Two, we examine IS and al-Qaeda statements and media publications addressing the pandemic to see whether there are any indications of new or heightened interest in attacking with biological materials or encouragement to followers to do so on their own.

In Chapter Three, we examine the groups' past interest in biological and chemical weapons. Although the groups showed interest in chemical and biological weapons prior to the pandemic, a short review of their experience provides a baseline for assessing what they might try or accomplish in the future.

In Chapter Four, we outline a few policy measures for authorities to consider that enhance capabilities to address naturally occurring pandemics and help deter, detect, and respond to the intentional use of biological agents for an attack.

In the concluding chapter, we explore explanations for why these two militant Islamic groups have not, thus far, opted to develop and use biological materials as a means of violence. Their statements and actions point to other means and potential targets to monitor closely. Any noteworthy change in their statements about the pandemic or a newfound fascination with poison, disease, or bacteria as weapon materials would be worrisome. In a pre-9/11 interview, Osama Bin Laden claimed that al-Qaeda had "chemical and nuclear weapons as a deterrent and if America used them against us, we reserve the right to use them."[26] Ayman Zawahiri, who was

---

[26] Osama Bin Laden quoted in Commission on the Intelligence Capabilities of the United States Regarding Weapons of Mass Destruction, Report to the President of the United States, March 31, 2005, p. 277.

al-Qaeda's second-in-command and who trained as a medical doctor, allegedly investigated the development of chemical and biological weapons and outlined what the group needed to do to develop these weapon capabilities.[27] Although stamping out these groups and those they inspire is not likely in the near term, some of the policy measures outlined in Chapter Four are designed to reduce the prospect of terrorists acquiring and using biological materials as weapons—and, if that does occur, to ensure that public health responses are effective at limiting the consequences.

Research Method and Sources

To assess whether the IS and al-Qaeda will pursue biological weapons in the wake of the pandemic, we based our analysis on a review of primary source literature produced by the two groups. Primary source materials were identified by various Site Intelligence Group databases; Aymenn Jawad Al-Tamimi's blog posts, which provides translations of significant Islamist group materials; and materials that we collected during field visits. A comparative exegesis of group statements contributed to a comparison of the groups' worldviews during the initial months of the pandemic and the messages they communicated to their followers. We confined our examination of primary source material to items that were publicly available. We did not examine social media data that were restricted or had limited distribution, except to the extent that they were referenced in secondary scholarly source material.

Additionally, we analyzed government, scholarly, and secondary source materials examining the groups' reactions to the pandemic as it unfolded. Secondary source material was obtained by searches for articles using the RAND Corporation's Online Catalogue System (ROCS), the ProQuest database, Google Scholar, and a private listserv composed of chemical and biological weapon experts, medical doctors, former diplomats, and military officials. These sources provided for a "snowball" approach, in which every source provided references to some new sources over the course of the project. This method of obtaining and examining source material entailed an iterative pro-

---

[27] Alan Cullison, "Inside Al-Qaeda's Hard Drive: Budget Squabbles, Baby Pictures, Office Rivalries—and the Path to 9/11," *The Atlantic*, September 2004.

cess in which each new source expanded our understanding of the qualitative issues examined and led to a regular reexamination of source material previously studied. These sources covered group motivations, demonstrated capabilities, societal vulnerabilities, and circumstances that ease weapon acquisitions and opportunities for conducting attacks. Sorting through primary sources, analytic assessments, and news reports provided a basis for us to employ a ground theory approach to source materials and render qualitative judgments on the central question as to whether the COVID-19 pandemic will stimulate these two groups to pursue biological weapons.

As part of our look at the motivations and capabilities of the groups, we also outline why they have not opted to pursue biological weapons. Far too often, analysis of terrorist threats focuses on what analysts think might be possible rather than on the empirical record. Although it is essential to consider the possibility of developments that have never occurred, it is also valuable to consider why something does *not* happen under favorable conditions. Understanding what prevents something from occurring helps to identify bulwarks that need to be strengthened. Finally, thinking about a threat from multiple perspectives ensures a calibrated assessment.

Given the difficulty that many national governments have had responding to the pandemic, it is natural for analysts to conclude that the IS, al-Qaeda, and those they inspire might see vulnerabilities to exploit in the future. Our analysis weighs arguments and counterarguments about the prospects of militant Islamic groups pursuing biological weapons, highlighting the value of policy measures that will not only help with future natural outbreaks but also improve capabilities to deter, counter, and/or respond to an intentional use of biological materials as weapons.

CHAPTER TWO

Pandemic Narratives of the Islamic State and al-Qaeda: Blessing a Deadly Means?

The Islamic State's Pandemic Narrative

When U.S. forces, North Atlantic Treaty Organization (NATO) allies, Kurdish fighters, Iranian-supported militias, and Iraqi forces retook Mosul from the IS in 2017, the remaining adherents of the group slipped away into the desert areas around the Euphrates valley. In many ways, these fugitives were thus naturally isolated and socially distanced when COVID-19 swept the globe. Nonetheless, as countries in Asia, Europe, and North America issued lockdown orders and other mandatory health guidance in March 2020 in response to the pandemic, the IS and al-Qaeda also counseled their followers.

The IS issued guidance in *al-Naba*—its official media outlet—via a text-laden infographic containing "Shari'i directives to deal with the epidemics."[1] The publication urged readers to put their trust in "the authority of Anas (may God be pleased with him) that the Prophet used to say: 'Oh God, I seek refuge in You from leprosy, madness, and from the malaise of illnesses.'"[2] The *al-Naba* commentary encouraged people to stay away from lands afflicted with the virus and to stay in place. In essence, the IS told its followers not to travel.

---

[1] Translated and quoted in Aymenn Jawad Al-Tamimi, "Islamic State Advice on Coronavirus Pandemic," blog post, March 12, 2020a.

[2] Translated and quoted in Al-Tamimi, 2020a.

In contrast to previous statements by IS leaders and in publications encouraging followers to take their fight to Europe and the United States, *al-Naba* urged that the "healthy should not enter the land of the epidemic and the afflicted should not exit."[3] This stay-in-place guidance echoed the travel restrictions announced by governments all around the globe. Many of the approximately 16,000 IS fighters and 65,000 family members had either gone into hiding in the Syrian and Iraqi desert areas or remained in detention camps in Syrian and Iraqi border areas.[4]

The guidance to those who contracted the virus was also to stay in place. These instructions are counterintuitive for a group of people who regularly organize suicide bombings and suicide attacks. To weaponize COVID-19, one might expect the IS to instead encourage its followers to become superspreaders. But, thus far, this has not happened. Sickened individuals are urged to stay in place and avoid spreading the disease.

As the pandemic took on global proportions and U.S. and coalition forces continued to withdraw from the region, IS members who remained stepped up their war-zone activities to influence and extort locals and to conduct attacks on military and police facilities. The IS message to those who remained in the Syria-Iraq region is to be patient and ready themselves to take advantage of the pandemic circumstances because it is the work of Allah. The initial impact of the pandemic—regardless of the extent of its spread—was to slow movement and activities of all kinds, including those of IS fighters.

One IS publication stated that "the plague" was not the result of a lab accident or a creation of nature, but an act of God to punish crusaders and apostates. An article in *al-Naba* opined that

> [the] torment [is] sent by God on Whomsoever He wills, and God has made it a mercy for the believers. Whosoever dwells in his land patient and awaiting as the plague fall[s] know[s] that it will only strike one

---

[3] *Al-Naba* quoted in Rashmee Roshan Lall, "In Time of Coronavirus, ISIS Shows Method in Its Murderous Madness," *The Arab Weekly*, March 22, 2020.

[4] Andrew Hanna, "Islamists Imprisoned Across the Middle East," Woodrow Wilson Center, June 24, 2021.

for whom God has decreed . . . [and they will receive] the reward of a martyr.[5]

As with so many aspects of radical interpretations of the Abrahamic religious traditions, it is a deterministic God that seals one's fate. Believers will be spared, but if a believer is stricken with the disease, it is God's determination to make them a martyr. The narrative argues that the areas most affected were the so-called enemies of Islam, such as the Chinese government, Shiites, Westerners, and apostate leaders in Muslim lands. As COVID-19 cases spread in China, Italy, the United States, the United Kingdom and France, IS adherents had their proof of Allah's vengeance on the enemies of Islam.

IS publications also provided health guidance asserting that this wisdom had divine origins. God's guidance was for each follower to "place his hand or clothing on his mouth when he sneezed" and when he "wakes from sleep, let him not dip his hand into the vessels until he washes three times, for he does not know where his hand spent the night."[6] To think about one's hand spending the night somewhere other than attached to one's body is oddly poetic, but the general guidance is to wash hands and do so thoroughly. The guidance for IS followers (and everyone else in the world, for that matter) was the same.

A week after these directives appeared, *al-Naba* published an editorial with a detailed assessment of the pandemic's implications that covered many different aspects of how the global pandemic affected the United States and other Western countries. Notably, it mentioned economic hardships resulting from lockdown orders; protests and riots that occurred in response to police killings of African-Americans during the pandemic; climate disasters, such as the West Coast fires; and restrictions on military operations and travel around the globe.[7] *Al-Naba* followed developments in the United States and Europe carefully and pivoted to a new narrative to justify the righteousness of the IS worldview.

---

[5] Translated and quoted in Al-Tamimi, 2020a.

[6] Translated and quoted in Al-Tamimi, 2020a.

[7] Translated and quoted in Aymenn Jawad Al-Tamimi, "Islamic State Editorial on the Coronavirus Pandemic," blog post, March 19, 2020b.

What is noteworthy about this mercurial shift to current events is that there is not a fascination with circumstances resulting from COVID-19 but rather a directing of attention to the latest trouble bedeviling the American people. In a later edition of *al-Naba*, an editorial entitled "The Worst Nightmares of the Crusaders" sent the following message:

> [F]ear of the epidemic among them has done more than what the epidemic itself has done, for their abodes have been shut, their markets and activities suspended, and many of them confined to their homes. And they have become on the verge of a great economic catastrophe. We ask God to increase their torment and save the believers from all that.[8]

Fear of the pandemic, the IS alleged, was doing more to disrupt the lives of the modern-day crusaders than the disease itself. The editorial seems to be saying that the economic might of the industrialized powers that seemingly influence the lives of Muslims is on the verge of collapse as a result of cowardice. The editorial urged Muslims to show "no pity for the disbelievers and the apostates even as they are at the height of their tribulation . . . and they must intensify the pressure on them so they become . . . incapable of harming Muslims."[9] The message was that the more that the perceived oppressors suffer, the less likely it is that they will harm Muslims.

The IS media also puts the plight of imprisoned IS followers into context. Concern about imprisoned adherents is a recurring theme; it is their version of "no one left behind." The IS worldview is contradictory, however, because the virus has crippled IS enemies while also threatening IS followers who are vulnerable to the disease—especially imprisoned IS fighters or IS followers housed in cramped conditions in refugee camps. Issuing calls to free Muslim prisoners is a long-standing practice intended to bolster the spirits of the imprisoned and their family members who long for their liberation.

Al-Naba implores believers to free their brethren from prisons. The March 19, 2020, *al-Naba* editorial explained that Muslims not only have an obligation "to protect themselves and their people from the spreading disease" but must "strive also to free the Muslim prisoners in the prisons of the idola-

---

[8] Translated and quoted in Al-Tamimi, 2020b.

[9] Translated and quoted in Al-Tamimi, 2020b.

ters and the camps of humiliation in which they are threatened by disease in addition to subjugation, coercion, hunger and enmity against themselves and their religion that they face from the idolaters."[10] In the Hasaka prison in Syria, which houses 4,000–5,000 hardened IS fighters in cramped conditions, protests have erupted concerning the potential spread of COVID-19 among the prisoners.[11] These protests served to remind those on the outside of the plight of those imprisoned. Iraqi authorities strengthened security at prisons housing IS prisoners for fear of attacks on those facilities.

Furthermore, according to a United Nations source, Kurdish fighters have almost 62,000 people in the Al-Hol refugee camp, approximately 25 miles southeast from Hasaka, which could suffer from a COVID-19 outbreak given the cramped and unsanitary conditions.[12] Many people in this camp are either IS refugees or persons displaced by conflict leading to the collapse of the IS.

Al-Qaeda's Pandemic Narrative

In March 2020, al-Qaeda issued a statement on the pandemic entitled "The Way Forward: A Word of Advice on the Coronavirus Pandemic" that sought to provide (1) context on the pandemic sweeping the globe and (2) guidance to followers and infidels alike.[13] Addressing a global audience, the document's authors observed that "As we all know, the coronavirus pandemic has cast its gloomy, painful shadow over the entire world" and suggested that al-Qaeda's duty was "to console our Muslim brothers and sisters and discuss the way forward for the Muslim World specifically and humanity in

---

[10] Translated and quoted in Al-Tamimi, 2020b.

[11] Eric Schmitt, "ISIS Prisoners Threaten U.S. Mission in Northeastern Syria, *New York Times*, May 25, 2020.

[12] The number of detainees in the Al-Hol camp fluctuates over time and according to the source but is consistently reported as more than 60,000. See Human Rights Watch, "Thousands of Foreigners Unlawfully Held in NE Syria," March 23, 2021; and United Nations, "UNICEF Urges Repatriation of All Children in Syria's Al-Hol Camp Following Deadly Fire," *UN News*, February 28, 2021.

[13] Al-Qaeda, "The Way Forward: A Word of Advice on the Coronavirus Pandemic," statement, March 31, 2020.

general."[14] This implies that the audience is not just followers or fellow Muslims, but the whole of humanity.[15] This narrative is more worldly, caring, and less vengeful than the IS's statements.

Al-Qaeda leaders clearly followed the global reaction to the pandemic and the emergency lockdown measures that countries worldwide took in mid-March 2020. Confirmation on how closely they followed events in the United States and other Western countries appears in the detail of their statement about the economic implications of the lockdowns. "In a matter of a few weeks, 4 million American have been left jobless . . . . The American economy has suddenly, and most unexpectedly, found itself in the [intensive care unit], in desperate need of a ventilator to resuscitate it, much like the Corona patients in the hospitals of New York."[16] Here, the statement makes a figurative connection between people sickened by COVID-19 and the economic freefall that resulted once a national emergency was announced and lockdown orders were issued.

A further indication of how closely al-Qaeda followed developments in the United States is that the statement points out that the "injection of funds into the economy amounts to a whopping 6 trillion dollars" and "this tremendous sum of money equals American losses in the two wars waged against the Muslim Ummah during the last two decades."[17] Linking the economic costs of the pandemic to the cost of two wars against al-Qaeda in Afghanistan and Iraq implies that the pandemic is an equivalent punishment for the wars. A connection is made between the impact or cost of military operations in Afghanistan and Iraq and the cost to the U.S. economy resulting from increased health care demands and an abrupt cessation of economic activities during the national emergency. In this view, the war has silently and invisibly shifted from Iraq, Syria, and Afghanistan to the metropolises of al-Qaeda's adversaries.

Al-Qaeda describes the pandemic as Allah's punishment of the West but also says it is "A General Call for the Masses in the Western World to

---

[14] Al-Qaeda, 2020.

[15] Al-Qaeda, 2020.

[16] Al-Qaeda, 2020.

[17] Al-Qaeda, 2020.

Embrace Islam." The pandemic is described as the "invisible soldier" with the power to threaten "the brittleness and vulnerability of your material strength."[18] Criticizing "technological achievement and globalization" the statement observes that "if someone sneezes in China, those in New York suffer from its consequences."[19] The wealthy oppressor nations are linked and the "invisible" or "divine" force is punishing those nations that are connected thematically by being oppressors of Muslims.

The statement goes on to proselytize "that we would like to introduce you to Islam" and reminds "non-Muslims to utilize their time in quarantine for finding out more about Islam from authentic sources."[20] The unprecedented nature of the global pandemic weighs on the writer of the statement, who describes how, "Today, humanity has become trapped in a darkness . . . . We must turn this calamity into a cause for unity in our ranks."[21] For al-Qaeda, this statement is oddly magnanimous. It raises the question whether this narrative line reflects a collective fear stemming from the uncertainties associated with the pandemic at the time or charts a new outlook on how to gain followers.

Highlighting Islam's relevance to the health challenges that the pandemic posed, the statement notes that "Islam is a hygiene-oriented Religion."[22] Central to the al-Qaeda religious narrative is the "importance of hygiene and cleanliness for preventing disease" and how "warding off viruses manifests itself in several facets of Islam."[23] For example, "anyone who finds himself in an area infected by a viral disease must not leave that area or travel to any other region, town, or village lest the infection spreads to new localities."[24] They are saying that sheltering in place reduces the likelihood of spreading the disease, saves lives, and bestows on the individual a reward that equals "that of a martyr because of his choice to preserve and protect

---

[18] Al-Qaeda, 2020.

[19] Al-Qaeda, 2020.

[20] Al-Qaeda, 2020.

[21] Al-Qaeda, 2020.

[22] Al-Qaeda, 2020.

[23] Al-Qaeda, 2020.

[24] Al-Qaeda, 2020.

human life."[25] This pious rhetoric contrasts with the many deadly attacks that al-Qaeda perpetrated in the late 1990s in East Africa and on 9/11 or those attacks that al-Qaeda inspired and/or heralded in London, Riyadh, Bali, Berlin, and Mumbai.

In contrast to this benevolent depiction of the Muslim who becomes a martyr by protecting others from the spread of infection by self-isolating, Western leaders are described as "least concerned about the health of the societies they are for. Instead of ensuring the provision of health facilities and medical supplies—some of which are inexpensive and simple, such as face masks and other personal protective equipment—they are obsessed with supplies of war and the tool of human eradication."[26] Al-Qaeda's view at the outset of the pandemic stressed the superiority of its worldview over that of Western leaders. This narrative was pitched at a grand level to serve as an alternative to the globalist view the organization associates with Western countries.

Similarities and Differences Between These Narratives

Both the IS and al-Qaeda narratives describe the pandemic as the work of Allah sent to punish the West for its wars in Afghanistan and Iraq, China for its suppression of the Uyghurs, Iran because Shiites are viewed by Sunnis as Islamic heretics, and the apostate Sunni Muslim regimes in Saudi Arabia, Egypt, Jordan, and the Gulf States. Speaking directly to these communities, al-Qaeda offered, "We have a brief message for the oppressive Crusaders and their hirelings among the Zionists and apostates: The fear and panic that has struck you is a good omen for us. We ask Allah to demonstrate His powers in your suffering and hasten your doom."[27] As previously discussed, the IS publication *al-Naba* asserts that

---

[25] Al-Qaeda, 2020.

[26] Al-Qaeda, 2020.

[27] Al-Qaeda, 2020.

> God Almighty has imposed something of His painful torment on the nations of His creation, most of them—and praise be to God—being of the idolaters, for fear of the epidemic among them has done more than what the epidemic itself has done, for their abodes have been shut, their markets and activities suspended, and many of them confined to their homes. We ask God to increase their torment and save the believers from all that.[28]

Both narratives view the economic damage to the West as a means of punishing the West for its oppression of Muslims.

The narratives of both groups contain discussion of hygienic measures central to Islamic tradition that Muslims should follow to protect themselves and others from the virus. However, there is also vague guidance about turning COVID-19 into a weapon to use against so-called non-believers, crusaders, apostates, heretics, or Zionists. As the pandemic continues to ebb and flow around the globe and the guidance on Islamic hygienic practices are repeated and embraced, this might serve to reinforce the idea that disease or biological materials are not legitimate weapons.

The narratives diverge on the apparent scope of how the groups perceive their audiences. The IS narrative is for those drawn to the idea of the IS and focuses on punishing infidels. There is no discussion about nonbelievers studying Islam while they are quarantined. There are no calls to save humanity. The IS's narrative and actions reveal a belief that the pandemic creates opportunities to attack enemies with the blessing of Allah. One can only speculate about a different explanation. By contrast (and despite its history of violence), al-Qaeda's narrative pitches its religious arguments to both Muslim and Western audiences by inviting the audience to learn about Islam. In several instances, the al-Qaeda narrative even seems to proselytize to non-Muslims. This contrast in content and tone might reveal a generational difference in how the two groups reacted to the pandemic. Alternatively, the differences might be geared to different perceptions of Muslim audiences. The IS narrative is unyielding, aggressive, and vindictive. The al-Qaeda narrative seems to embrace both a concern for the implications of

---

[28] Translated and quoted in Al-Tamimi, 2020b.

the pandemic and the idea that a more accommodating view is appreciated by everyone under the yoke of the pandemic.

The logic contained in both narratives is internally contradictory and provides different rationales for people to embrace. One analysis insightfully describes the elements of these narratives as a "diverse, and, often internally inconsistent, blend of communications including conspiracy theories, claims of the God's vengeance against its enemies, exhortation to weaponize the virus, and taking advantage of society's weakness by launching widespread attacks wherever and whenever possible."[29] In the view of these groups, the virus is both Allah's divine punishment of those who have not followed the faith and an attack on the perceived enemies of Islam.

As with many narratives from Islamic extremists, there is a profound sense of grievance and victimhood. The profound grievance is a consistent justification to attack those who are believed to have harmed Muslims. Whether it is suicide attacks or the invisible but deadly spread of COVID-19, conducting revenge on those who have harmed the Muslims is a legitimate justification. Ascribing the pandemic to Allah to killing the "crusaders and heretics" attempts to lend legitimacy to the violent acts of IS and al-Qaeda members and those they inspire.

After May 2020, references to COVID-19 generally disappeared from the narratives of both organizations. Instead, they focused on other topics, such as faltering economies, racial strife, forest fires, and other effects of climate change. The media organs of both groups also discussed recent terrorist attacks around the globe. The lack of attention to COVID-19 might have the consequence of reducing interest in the disease as means of punishment. Perhaps the new view is that COVID-19 is just one thing among many punishing the enemies of Islam.

---

[29] Arie W. Kruglanski, Rohan Gunaratna, Molly Ellenberg, and Anne Speckhard, "Terrorism in Time of the Pandemic: Exploiting Mayhem," *Global Security: Health, Science and Policy*, Vol. 5, No. 1, October 2020, p. 122.

Has the Pandemic Suppressed Attacks by the Islamic State and al-Qaeda?

Given the pandemic's second and third waves across North America and Europe in the autumn of 2020 and the winter and spring of 2021 and the disease's spread in South Asia, Latin America, and Africa, it is worth considering whether COVID-19 will return in similar or new ways as a topic in the worldview of the IS and al-Qaeda. Will the spread of disease in the Middle East, Africa, and South Asia (regions where violent Islamic extremists are operating) influence these groups' choices of weapons, attack plans, and global narratives? Will the spread of COVID-19 in these regions increase or diminish the idea of using biological materials as weapons? As of this writing, these groups have not mentioned the possibility of such an approach in their statements on the pandemic. Given that fact and the groups' spotty historical records of bioterrorism, it seems unlikely that such an approach will be pursued.

National lockdowns might have a chilling effect on militant activities of all kinds. Restrictions on travel and commerce has made insurgent movement more difficult. Increased public health protection measures have been implemented to contend with the spread of the virus and heighten preparations to handle disease outbreaks. The much-anticipated development of the COVID-19 vaccine highlighted the medical means to thwart the spread of the virus. These increased protective measures and widespread vaccinations might demonstrate to nonstate actors that using viruses as biological weapons are not certain to produce deadly results, unlike attacks that involve explosives. The delayed and uncertain results of biological weapons might, over time, diminish the fascination for IS and al-Qaeda members.

Some analysts have argued that inspired individuals might take it on themselves to wage attacks, as occurred in Europe. Thus far, these individual attacks have been carried out with conventional means; there have been only a few cases in which people not associated with militant Islamic groups acted as human virus delivery vehicles. At the beginning of the outbreak, a few isolated incidents occurred in which people spat on food or otherwise claimed to spread the disease. These incidents were few and largely inconsequential.[30] Right-wing extremists in the United States and Europe encouraged followers who contract the disease to seek out synagogues or crowds of Jewish people to infect.[31] There is no similar encouraging of members to conduct this type of attack in IS or al-Qaeda pandemic narratives. Rather, as Koblentz and Kiesel note, "Jihadist groups have treated the pandemic primarily as an opportunity for propaganda and recruiting."[32]

Using humans as delivery vehicles for disease has frequently been a concern, but cases are rare and not significant. A suicide bombing is an effective and readily available alternative that these groups consistently use with lethal, immediate, and dramatic results. By contrast, infecting others with a virus that entails a delay and is not always lethal lacks the same punch. Thus far, there are no publicly known cases of an IS or al-Qaeda member sickened with a lethal disease acting as a human delivery vehicle of infection.

---

[30] Lucia Binding, "Coronavirus: Two Charged with Terror Offenses over Threats to Spread COVID-19, "*Sky News*, April 10, 2020.

[31] Kruglanski et al., 2020, p. 127. For an extensive examination of right-wing interest in biological agents as weapons, see Ely Karmon, *The Radical Right's Obsession with Bioterrorism*, Israel: International Institute for Counter-Terrorism, June 2020.

[32] Koblentz and Kiesel, 2021, p. 10.

CHAPTER THREE

Past Attacks Reveal Limitations on Future Interest and Use of Biological Weapons

The IS and al-Qaeda pandemic narratives do not reveal a new or heightened interest in using the virus or any other biological material as a weapon. Instead, the IS, al-Qaeda, and affiliated and inspired groups have sought to take advantage of restrictions that the pandemic has caused. Attacks by Islamic militants via conventional means have continued in war zones where counterterrorism security forces have retreated because of the pandemic or broader policy shifts. As some scholars have noted, the retraction of security forces has been an "accelerant" to these attacks rather than a pure cause of them.[1] Yet, even in these areas, the ebb and flow of the threat these attacks pose has thus far been manageable for national and international coalition counterterrorism forces.

Outside the war zones in Syria, Iraq, and Afghanistan, the pace of attacks has been steady. Violent Islamists have continued a series of attacks in Southeast Asia. In many ways, Africa has become the new frontline. Activities of locally focused groups that align with the IS or al-Qaeda brands have flourished in Nigeria, Mali, and Mozambique. However, the weapons and modes of operations are traditional strikes with conventional means. Although these operations have been deadly and gruesome, they have not involved COVID-19 or biological materials. Nor have there

---

[1] Michael Knights and Alex Almeida, "Remaining and Expanding: The Recovery of Islamic State Operations in Iraq in 2019-2020," *CTC Sentinel*, Vol. 13, No. 5, May 2020, p. 27.

been any significant or sustained rhetoric urging the use of COVID-19 as a weapon.

U.S. and NATO security forces have left or been repositioned in Syria, Iraq, and Afghanistan and are not likely to return in great numbers unless there is an urgent need. The short-term result is that insurgent groups, predominantly the IS and those aligned with or inspired by it, have taken advantage of the reduction in security operations to conduct attacks on garrisoned security forces and to extend their influence in new or previously held areas.

To anticipate the types of tactics that the IS and al-Qaeda might use, it is instructive to examine their previous attempts: the IS's development and use of chemical agents and al-Qaeda's efforts to develop biological weapons. In both cases, these groups operated in territorial sanctuaries for years, recruited individuals with technical skills specifically to develop chemical and biological weapons, but had only limited success with crude chemical agents when all was said and done. Both groups also moved on to conventional means of violence that were easier to produce and deliver and that achieved the desired deadly results. Despite rhetorical claims of desires to use biological weapons, research on them, and limited use of them, the IS and al-Qaeda instead conducted many attacks via deadly conventional means, such as suicide bombings, knifings, shootings, and driving vehicles into crowds of people. Interest in such exotic means as biological and chemical agents as weapons was transient and not an obsession for either group.

Islamic State Use of Chemical Agents Might Reveal Limits on Pursuit of Biological Weapons

To assess whether members of the IS will be inspired to pursue infectious biological weapons as a means of violence in the wake of the pandemic, it is useful to examine their history of using unconventional weaponry. Although the publicly available evidence of IS members pursuing biological weapons is scant, they do have a track record of using industrial chemicals and producing sulfur mustard agent as weapons.[2] Examining the group's experience with

---

[2] Joby Warrick, "ISIS Used Chemical Weapons on Iraqi Prisoners, U.N. Investigators Find," *Washington Post*, May 13, 2021. This news story reports on a UN report that

chemical weapons serves as a useful, albeit imperfect, surrogate for its inclination and potential success in developing and using biological weapons.

When the IS took over large swaths of eastern Syria and western Iraq, it had personnel with technical skills, access to laboratories, deadly materials, and desires to kill adversaries indiscriminately to redress its grievances and protect its formation of a state. Although it did not pursue biological weapons, it did acquire and use toxic industrial chemicals. It also developed, produced, and used a crude sulfur mustard agent. Publicly available sources state that the IS used chlorine and sulfur mustard somewhere between 37 and 76 times.[3] Although this is a disquieting fact, a short examination of IS development and use of chemical agents as weapons helps calibrate what the group might be able to do with biological materials as weapons. IS technical capabilities to use chlorine as a weapon were minimal and the sulfur mustard produced was of a low grade and not particularly effective. Given the sanctuary and capabilities that IS possessed in Syria and Iraq from June 2014 to January 2017, it is noteworthy that the use of toxic industrial chemicals and low-grade sulfur mustard agent proved much less deadly than many of the conventional means they used.

For the IS, the use of chemical agents produced some casualties in short order and might have kept Kurdish fighters at bay, but these weapons were difficult to deploy with much accuracy and proved largely unsuccessful in producing significant casualties. Kurdish fighters noted that the use of chemical agents did produce fear in their troops, but actual casualties were much less than those caused by conventional weaponry. In contrast, if the

accuses the IS of genocide. The UN report refers to the IS testing nicotine (a toxin) on Iraqi prisoners. Although a disturbing revelation, this is a report of testing the effects of a noninfectious material and not a full weapon.

[3] According to Strack, the IHS Markit's Conflict Monitor open-source dataset lists 76 uses of chemicals from June 2014 to October 2017. See Columb Strack, "The Evolution of the Islamic State's Chemical Weapons Effort," *CTC Sentinel*, Vol. 10, No. 9, October 2017, p. 19. The University of Maryland group chose to limit its analysis to sulfur mustard attacks because "reports on mustard agent attacks are better supported due to the potential to test for specific breakdown products in biological or soil samples" (Markus K. Binder, Jillian M. Quigley, and Herbert F. Tinsley, "Islamic State Chemical Weapons: A Case Contained by Its Context?" *CTC Sentinel*, Vol. 11, No. 3, March 2018, p. 27).

IS used biological agents on a battlefield or a non-war-zone environment, the effects would not be immediate and the accuracy and effectiveness would be similarly challenging. Additionally, medical treatments—such as antibiotics or vaccines—might be available to mitigate the effectiveness of biological agents. Although the ongoing pandemic has stretched the public health resources of many countries to capacity, it is likely that capabilities to respond to outbreaks of communicable diseases will improve worldwide as a result of the COVID-19 pandemic. Augmenting capabilities to detect and address natural outbreaks of disease will provide some dual-use benefits that will improve capabilities to manage terrorist use of some biological weapons. Improved disease surveillance and communication between health care authorities will detect both natural outbreaks and intentionally caused events more quickly. Better preparation for handling natural large-scale disease outbreaks will improve health care providers' abilities to handle intentional uses of biological agents. Countermeasures and treatments developed for specific biological agents will be effective in addressing commonly known warfare agents, but it is difficult to predict which biological agents might be used. Consequently, improvements in general capabilities to handle widespread disease outbreaks are important. In the future, biological agents commonly envisioned for military pursuits might not be the weapon of choice for nonstate actors, who frequently improvise with what they have an opportunity to acquire and use.[4] Developing broad-spectrum detection and response capabilities might prove more valuable over time.

The IS progression from loading munitions with chlorine to loading them with low-grade sulfur mustard agent represents some organizational learning and improvement in IS technical capabilities. From June 2015 until spring 2016, the IS conducted its chemical attacks in Syria and Iraq. In the early days, the IS used widely available industrial chemicals, such as chlorine and phosphine, in simple delivery devices, such as roadside or vehicle-borne improvised explosive devices. In summer 2016 and beyond, an IS cell produced low-grade sulfur mustard agent and delivered it in mortar shells and improvised rockets. The final phase of IS use of mustard agent

---

[4] John Parachini, "Putting WMD Terrorism into Perspective," *Washington Quarterly*, Vol. 26, No. 4, Autumn 2003.

saw extensive U.S. bombing of suspected IS chemical cells. There were a few sporadic attacks in January 2017, then nothing.[5]

Over the course of the nearly three years when the IS controlled large portions of Syria and Iraq, IS use of chemicals as a battlefield weapon did evolve and advance, but only slightly. The extent of the IS's chemical weapons development was very modest considering that it controlled territory and had access to chemicals, a large personnel base for identifying people with scientific and engineering skills, some individuals who has been junior employees in Saddam Hussein's chemical weapon program, and laboratory equipment in Mosul. There is no publicly available evidence that the IS explored biological weapons.

The IS's use of chemical agents in war zones in Syria and Iraq was a disquieting development, but concern should be tempered by the limited nature of their use, the low number of casualties, and the failure to use these agents effectively when facing imminent defeat in Mosul. IS use of chlorine and mustard agents was generally crude and ineffective. In contrast, the IS's procurement of drones was more successful: The adaptations made to deliver explosives were new, widely used and effective, and they proliferated to theaters of operations outside the Middle East.[6] Some have argued that these drone attacks provide a psychological effect similar to that of attacks with chemical agents, as well as being more deadly.[7]

What remains puzzling about the IS's use of chlorine and mustard agents is that the group never took credit for their use. Using chemical agents—poison—as a weapon is prohibited by the Chemical Weapons Convention and widely viewed as taboo by the international community. This raises the question of whether whoever in the IS was involved in the use of chemical weapons feared breaking that taboo. Sixteen issues of *al-Naba* at the time of the chemical attacks did not mention a single use of chemical agents. The IS did all manner of grisly things prior to the alleged use of chemical agents and did not hesitate to post videos of horrific beheadings, mass executions,

---

[5] Strack, 2017.

[6] Don Rassler, *The Islamic State and Drones: Supply, Scale, and Future Threats*, West Point, N.Y.: Combating Terrorism Center, July 2018.

[7] Strack, 2017, pp. 21–22.

or burning a captive alive.[8] The IS does not shy away from cruel and inhuman violence and publicizing it widely. So, why not shout to the world that it used chemical agents in combat?

One possible explanation is that the IS members involved felt the impact of their message was effectively communicated by the use of the weapon. There was no need to claim credit. Another explanation might be that the IS members involved in the attack were mired in combat and did not have a good way to communicate with the organization's propaganda wing. Alternatively, these members might have feared that taking credit would weaken their operational security, cause someone in their ranks to be repulsed by the chemical attacks, and leak information that would lead to a punishing attack—and bombing attacks by U.S. forces is what eventually seemed to stop IS use of chemical agents. Finally, although not as likely, it is possible that even IS fighters, cognizant of the ramifications of the use of chemical agents, did not want to acknowledge that they had used them. Whatever the explanation is for the IS not taking credit for the use of chemical agents, it warrants further investigation because it might reveal important insights regarding how to dissuade other nonstate actors from using these types of weapons. Explanations for why terrorists do or do not claim credit have not been thoroughly or consistently examined in recent years. The few scholarly examinations of terrorist claims of credit have been insightful at the time of their writing, but there is a critical need to update the analysis with a focus on chemical weapons.[9]

Considering why the IS personnel who were responsible for producing and weaponizing chemical agents were reluctant to take credit is relevant for assessing whether the same players might seek to use biological agents as a weapon in the future. If they were reluctant to claim credit for a chemical attack that had immediate effect, would they be more satisfied with the delayed results of biological material, or less so? If victims or authorities were alerted that bacteria or viruses had been used as a weapon and there

---

[8] Binder, Quigley, and Tinsley, 2018, p. 29.

[9] Bruce Hoffman, "Why Terrorists Don't Claim Credit," *Terrorism and Political Violence*, Vol. 9, No. 1, Spring 1997. Also see Austin L. Wright, *Why Do Terrorists Claim Credit? Attack-Level and Country-Level Analyses of Factors Influencing Terrorist Credit-Taking Behavior*, Austin, Tex.: University of Texas at Austin, July 16, 2014.

was an effective medical response available, would terrorists be more likely to use explosives instead of biological weapons?

Explosives, bullets, machetes, or vehicles driven into crowds of people produce terrifying and immediate results in contrast to biological weapons. Biological agents used as weapons produce delayed death and, in many cases, the cause of illness or death is not immediately obvious. Biological agents, such as viruses and bacteria, used as weapons do not have the immediacy of explosions, mass shootings, and crushing people with vehicles. Additionally, there are antidotes and prophylactic measures that can be taken when use of a biological agent is discovered. In 2001, the people exposed to anthrax, a bacterial agent, were issued cipro, an antibiotic. Similarly, people can be vaccinated for many viral agents that might serve as biological weapons. Most toxins, in contrast, can produce deadly effects more rapidly and there are not always antidotes readily available. The limitation of toxins is that they are difficult to produce in enough volume and are difficult to disseminate effectively over a wide area. Thus, although biological agents cause great fear because of how they might be disseminated to affect a large population and cause a horrific form of death, countervailing features make this task difficult to accomplish and consequently make these agents less-attractive weapons for such nonstate actors as the IS.

Part of the challenge of discerning the IS's motives and capabilities is understanding who is being discussed. Too often, a broad brush depicts a group as a single actor rather than as individuals involved who come together as a group to do certain things. The IS under Abu Bakr al-Baghdadi's leadership clearly endorsed grotesque violence as a way of life. But it is unclear what the next generation of IS leaders perceive as the best means to further their worldview.

Al-Qaeda's Historical Interest in Biological Weapons Stalled

Reviewing elements of a group's effort provides a baseline for assessing whether members of the group might try to re-create an interest in biological weapons in the wake of the COVID-19 pandemic. With enough time, money, and personnel, terrorist groups will pursue a wide variety of attack options. Militant Islamic leaders have justified pursuing unconventional weapons and weapon materials since the 1990s. When these leaders have mentioned WMD, they did so because WMD were perceived as the most-powerful and most-feared weapon capabilities. Frequently, no meaningful distinction was made among chemical, biological, radiological, or nuclear weapons. In the late 1990s, al-Qaeda pursued biological weapons, but it was a crude and ultimately unsuccessful effort.

When al-Qaeda enjoyed the protection of the Taliban-controlled government of Afghanistan, they could investigate the development of exotic weapons. Videos of al-Qaeda agents killing dogs with chemical agents showed the group's interest in unconventional weapons but also revealed that its capabilities were crude. Zawahiri, al-Qaeda's second-in-command at the time, revealed that the group did not pursue biological materials as weapons until leaders saw how fearful U.S. officials seemed to be of an attack with biological weapons.[10] Apparently, once al-Qaeda leaders picked up on the widely publicized fears of U.S. officials, the group began to investigate biological agents at its Tarnak Farms compound in Kandahar, Afghanistan. Despite this interest and the availability of a few individuals with limited technical expertise, efforts did not get very far.

The 2005 report by the Commission on the Intelligence Capabilities of the United States Regarding Weapons of Mass Destruction noted that the "Intelligence Community concluded that at the time of the commencement of the war in Afghanistan, al-Qaida's biological weapon program was both more advanced and more sophisticated than analysts had previously assessed."[11] With passage of time, subsequent information about al-Qaeda's exploration of biological weapons led noted analyst W. Seth Carus to describe al-Qaeda's biological weapon program as "still in the formative stage in September 2001. Although the group had made progress in constructing a laboratory in Afghanistan, there is no evidence that it ever

---

[10] This material is drawn from a memo from Ayman Zawahiri to Muhammad Atef as cited in Cullison, 2004. Also see W. Seth Carus, *A Short History of Biological Warfare: From Pre-History to the 21st Century*, Washington, D.C.: Center for the Study of Weapons of Mass Destruction, Occasional Paper No. 12, August 2017, p. 43.

[11] Commission on the Intelligence Capabilities of the United States Regarding Weapons of Mass Destruction, 2005, pp. 269–270.

obtained any biological agents."[12] The 2005 commission drew a conclusion about what analysts had previously believed, but evidence gathered over time suggests that the program amounted to much less than previously anticipated. For example, despite possessing some commercial equipment that could be used for development and production of biological agents, the group's technical expertise was limited. Al-Qaeda operatives were not able to acquire the biological material needed to embark on the weaponization process. Successful efforts would have required more people with technical expertise, enough biological material to fashion into a weapon, and enough time to do so. Al-Qaeda leaders ultimately gave up on pursuing biological weapons and turned their attention to chemical weapons.[13]

What is noteworthy is that al-Qaeda could not obtain agent pathogens at any facility in Afghanistan or from abroad. Nor was it able to cultivate anthrax from naturally occurring sources in Afghanistan. Failure to accomplish these two steps might reflect on the quality of the personnel involved. At the request of Zawahiri, Hambali recruited Yazid Sufaat as having the expertise to advance al-Qaeda's efforts to prepare a biological weapon.[14] Sufaat only had a basic undergraduate education in general biological science with a concentration in clinical laboratory training at Sacramento State University. He had also served as a laboratory technician in the Malaysian military. He later set up a company to conduct drug tests for private companies. He was not a scientist with advanced academic training, nor was he a weapon engineer.[15]

---

[12] Carus, 2017, p. 43.

[13] Carus, 2017.

[14] Riduan Isamuddin, known as Hambili, was the operations chief of the Southeast Asian al-Qaeda affiliate Jamaah Islamiya. During interrogation, Hambali described being involved in al-Qaeda's effort to produce anthrax in Malaysia (Daniel Benjamin, "Terrorist Groups: The Quest for Apocalyptic Capabilities," in Kurt M. Campbell, ed., *The Challenge of Proliferation*, Queenstown, Md.: Aspen Strategy Group, 2005, p. 46). Also see Renè Pita and Rohan Gunaratna, "Revisiting Al-Qa'ida's Anthrax Program," *CTC Sentinel*, Vol. 2, No. 5, May 2009.

[15] Leitenberg, 2005, p. 30.

According to the 9/11 Commission, Sufaat did not start to work on producing a biological weapon for use by al-Qaeda until December 2000.[16] The WMD Commission reported a few years later that it appeared that al-Qaeda began work on biological materials in Afghanistan in 1999.[17] Al-Qaeda had one or two years to produce a biological weapon of some type and failed to do so. This outcome is not surprising given that some states worked for years with considerable resources and top-flight talent to develop biological weapons and still struggled.[18]

Relevant scientific talent is simply not enough to develop and produce biological weapons. Authors of a 2009 review of al-Qaeda's biological weapons activities observed that "what characterized al-Qa'ida's anthrax program were its unsuccessful attempts to recruit Pakistani and Indonesian scientists who had access to microbial culture collections."[19] Although access to biological material that is the feedstock for biological weapon production is critical, a combination of other things also need to come together for nonstate actors to develop, produce or procure, weaponize, and deliver biological or chemical materials that pose a threat comparable to recent conventional bombings.[20]

There are several possible explanations for why al-Qaeda's pursuit of biological agents did not advance before U.S. forces swept in, toppled the Taliban government that protected these al-Qaeda operatives, and chased them out of Afghanistan. First, some individuals in al-Qaeda had some biological science training but not nearly enough to procure the necessary ingredients, produce enough material, and weaponize it. These are all development and

---

[16] National Commission on Terrorist Attacks Upon the United States, *Final Report of the National Commission on Terrorist Attacks Upon the United States*, Washington, D.C., June 17, 2004, p. 151.

[17] Commission on the Intelligence Capabilities of the United States Regarding Weapons of Mass Destruction, 2005, pp. 269–270.

[18] For a discussion of the difficulty that states have had in developing biological weapons see Elisa D. Harris, "Threat Reduction and North Korea's CBW Program," *Nonproliferation Review*, Vol. 11, No. 3, Fall/Winter 2004.

[19] Pita and Gunaratna, 2009.

[20] This is a long-standing observation that is not always taken into account in the literature on nonstate actors and WMD. See John Parachini, "Comparing Motives and Outcomes of Mass Casualty Terrorism Involving Conventional and Unconventional Weapons," *Studies in Conflict & Terrorism*, Vol. 24, No. 5, 2001.

production tasks nation-states with substantial scientific infrastructure, scientific talent, and financial resources have taken years to accomplish—and not all have been successful.

Second, al-Qaeda grew out of an anti-Soviet insurgency movement dominated by individuals who had considerable experience with conventional weapons but little to no experience with exotic weapon materials, such as toxins, viruses, and bacteria. As Zawahiri noted, al-Qaeda explored the potential of biological weapons late in its evolution as a terrorist organization.[21] Following the 9/11 attacks and the rapid advance of U.S. personnel in Afghanistan, there was neither time nor adequate safe haven for the difficult development, production, and engineering processes required.

Third, al-Qaeda viewed exploring biological agents and chemicals to use as weapons as only part of a portfolio of means for killing. As with any portfolio of options, leaders go with what they are confident will achieve the desired outcome. Suicide bombers driving cars loaded with explosives into U.S. embassies in Kenya and Tanzania was not expected, but it was a proven tactic. Al-Qaeda took a modern means of everyday travel and turned it into a weapon of mass destruction. It did not require development and production of weapon material or complicated engineering to load the material into delivery means, such as mortar shells or short-range rockets.

Al-Qaeda's track record of conducting mass casualty attacks with conventional means is an indication that they turned to other methods when their effort to produce biological weapons stalled. The group has not posed anywhere near the level of threat it did before it was largely pushed out of Afghanistan and Osama bin Laden was killed. Al-Qaeda-aligned groups continue to operate around the globe, most prominently in Syria. On balance, as a global organization, it is a shadow of what it was when it had a sanctuary in Afghanistan. In the short to medium term, it seems unlikely that it will gain the opportunity, skills, and materials to embark on a biological weapons program even in the wake of the COVID-19 pandemic.

---

[21] Cullison, 2004.

Ricin Plots Show Capability Limits of Inspired Individuals

As already mentioned, the IS as an organization in Syria and Iraq is greatly weakened. As a concept, the group remains salient, and violent Islamic groups are affiliating or aligning with it in Africa, South Asia, and Southeast Asia. Although inspired to align with the IS, these groups wage attacks in their local domains with conventional weaponry. There have been no serious attempts to employ unconventional weapons, such as chemical or biological agents. The possibility that the IS, al-Qaeda, or those aligned with them might develop some biological agent capability in the future is not zero, but it is small. Conventional means are readily available and have repeatedly produced mass casualties.

Although the IS and al-Qaeda might not pursue biological agents in a concerted fashion, will inspired individuals take it on themselves to do so? Advances in biotechnology have led some analysts to argue that individuals could now do what was unimaginable in the past. Al-Qaeda, and then the IS, inspired many individuals to conduct attacks on their own. Vehicle attacks in Nice, London, and New York are examples. Some analysts have concerns about whether individuals inspired by the message of these groups will take it on themselves to engage in violence to carry out jihad as they interpret it. Might they, inspired by the COVID-19 pandemic, seek to use biological materials in such efforts? To evaluate this prospect, we examined past cases of inspired individuals who sought to produce the toxin ricin.

In analyzing these cases, we found that warnings about the extent of technological advances in the life sciences have, thus far, been exaggerated. None of these cases has amounted to much. They reveal motivations, but a lack of capability. Although ricin is a protein material, the challenge of obtaining enough of it and weaponizing it has proved formidable. The few ricin plots that have been attempted illustrate the limits that are encountered in pursuit of an exotic weapon material.

A few attempts have been made by individuals in the United States to produce ricin for use as a weapon; these efforts have been unsuccessful.[22] One

---

[22] George Smith, "The American Way of Bioterror—An A–Z of Ricin Crackpots: Homebrew Poison of Choice to the Hard of Thinking," *The Register*, April 22, 2008.

analyst describes the Americans who sought to produce ricin as "crackpot bean pounders."[23] They have generally been social outcasts who express grievances against others, frequently those in authority. Elsewhere, Islamic militants inspired by the IS and al-Qaeda have been only marginally more successful, but the result has been the same—a failed plot that was ineffective.

In 2003, British authorities broke up an alleged al-Qaeda cell in Wood Green, London, that was believed to be producing some type of poison for an attack. Ultimately, authorities arrested Kamel Bourgass, the mastermind of the cell, who was an Algerian national with alleged links to the Armed Islamic Group.[24] In the apartment raided by authorities, small piles of cherry stones, apple pips, and 22 castor beans were recovered.[25] The effort was amateurish; authorities believed Bourgass was following a recipe from *The Poisoner's Handbook* and using a coffee grinder to mill the beans to make ricin. Early reports suggested that the cell produced the toxin, but later reports indicated that forensic evidence revealed that ricin had not actually been produced.[26]

Fifteen years after the London case, German authorities in Cologne arrested Sief Allah H., an Egyptian who reportedly purchased castor beans via the internet with the intent of making ricin for an improvised explosive device.[27] In contrast to the London case, the perpetrator in the Cologne case amassed 3,000 castor beans and produced a small amount of powdery substance that tested positive for ricin. Like the London case, the perpetrator followed simple instructions using an electric coffee grinder to mill the beans, but this time the tutorial came via an instructional video on the

---

[23] Smith, 2008.

[24] Jay Edwards and Benoît Gomis, *Islamic Terrorism in the UK Since 9/11: Reassessing the "Soft" Response*, London: Chatham House, International Security Program Paper, ISP PP2011/03, June 2011.

[25] Jared Ahmad, "Serving the Same Interests: The Wood Green Ricin Plot, Media-State-Terror Relations and the 'Terrorism' *Dispotif*," *Media, War & Conflict*, Vol. 12, No. 4, 2019; Leitenberg, 2005.

[26] Brian Michael Jenkins and Joseph Trella, *Carnage Interrupted: An Analysis of Fifteen Terrorist Plots Against Public Surface Transportation*, San Jose, Calif.: Mineta Transportation Institute, Report 11-20, April 2012.

[27] Florian Flade, "The June 2018 Cologne Ricin Plot: A New Threshold in Jihadi Bio Terror," *CTC Sentinel*, Vol. 11, No. 7, August 2018.

internet. A combination of brushes with German local law enforcement and tips from British authorities enabled German authorities to apprehend Sief Allah H. before he could produce a significant quantity of the toxin. Flade describes this as "the first time a jihadi terrorist in the West successfully produced ricin." Nevertheless, to put this in perspective, Flade cites an interview with a German security official in concluding that weaponizing ricin in an improvised explosive device was regarded as very difficult.[28]

What distinguished the Cologne case from the London case is the means with which a lone actor could obtain materials over the internet and get clear instruction. But the steps needed to create enough material and fashion it into a weapon without endangering himself still eluded Sief Allah H. In the end, his effort was like those that preceded it—amateurish and unsuccessful.

Several factors make the use of biological materials as weapons very difficult for nonstate actors and thus predispose these actors to use other means to carry out their agendas. Milton Leitenberg, an analyst with decades of research on the subject of biological and chemical weapons, succinctly outlined

> five essential requirements [that] must be mastered in order to produce biological agents [are]:
>
> - One must obtain the appropriate strain of the disease pathogen.
> - One must know how to handle the organism correctly.
> - One must know how to grow it in a way that will produce the appropriate characteristics.
> - One must know how to store the culture, and to scale-up production properly.
> - One must know how to disperse the product properly.[29]

Failure to produce an effective biological weapon can occur at any one of these five steps. Mastering all these steps safely is a formidable task that even state weapon programs with considerable resources at their disposal have struggled to accomplish.

---

[28] Flade, 2018.

[29] Leitenberg, 2005, p. 46.

CHAPTER FOUR

Policy Measures to Reduce the Possibility of Bioterrorism in the Wake of the Pandemic

The risk of the IS or al-Qaeda successfully pursuing a biological weapon capability is a combination of threat, vulnerability, and the consequences that might result.[1] The threat is a combination of motivation, capabilities, and the opportunity that perpetrators have to assemble the capabilities (depending on availability of materials and their ability to forge them into effective weapons). As the COVID-19 pandemic has revealed, the consequence of an infectious disease outbreak—natural or intentionally caused—can be significant. Moreover, the difficulty that advanced industrial countries have had responding to the COVID-19 pandemic show the vulnerability of major countries—notably, the United States, the United Kingdom, Italy, Germany, Sweden, Brazil, Russia, and China.

However, not all biological agents present the same consequence as an infectious disease like COVID-19. An infectious virus presents a rapid effect in transmitting the disease from one person to another. In contrast, some bacterial agents or toxins pose less risk because the ability of a perpetrator to disseminate one of these biological agents to a wide population is limited, and the population likely to be affected is smaller than the population that an infectious disease might afflict.[2] Highly effective mass casualty attacks

---

[1] Henry H. Willis, "Guiding Resource Allocations Based on Terrorism Risk," Santa Monica, Calif.: RAND Corporation, WR-371-CTRMP, March 2006.

[2] Some bacterial agents cause infectious diseases. For example, strep throat, tuberculosis, and plague are caused by bacterial agents.

with bacterial agents or toxins require a sufficient volume of material and a means of dissemination that ensures inhalation or ingestion. There is a small probability of an actor disseminating these biological agents in a way that would effectively produce mass casualties—but if that step is effectively performed, it could lead to significant consequences.

There are many factors that influence the risk of nonstate actors using biological agents. Vulnerability to the effects of biological weapons and the potential consequences of that vulnerability are both important but highly variable factors. In the wake of the COVID-19 pandemic, countries will have built up some capabilities as a response to the pandemic and thus be less vulnerable to infectious disease outbreaks. These capabilities might also help countries to better manage the consequences of a biological weapon attack. Thus, a low-probability event might entail even fewer damaging consequences than would have been faced in the pre-pandemic period.

The threat of the IS and al-Qaeda using biological materials as weapons is much lower than the threat of alternative conventional means. However, given that the probability is not zero and that technological developments in the future might increase that probability, states need to take action to reduce the risks. Taking measures that address naturally occurring infectious disease outbreaks and are also relevant for unlikely (but possible) intentional biological weapon attacks will better position governments to address the overlapping aspects of these related but different threats.

The pandemic will certainly lead to better global public health practices and will likely reinforce the stance against the use of poison and disease as a terrorist means of killing. David Franz, former head of the U.S. Army Medical Research Institute of Infectious Diseases, has suggested that COVID-19 is the public health community's "mushroom cloud."[3] In the struggle to contain the pandemic and care for those afflicted, public health capabilities around the globe have been challenged like never before and health care providers are responding with varying degree of effectiveness. The consequences of the pandemic were worse in several countries where political leaders ignored the advice of health authorities for short-term political rea-

---

[3] David R. Franz, "Biological Security and Health in the Post-Pandemic World: The Infectious Disease Community's 'Mushroom Cloud'?" *CBW Magazine*, Vol. 13, No. 2, January–June 2020.

sons. It is to be hoped that the effects of the pandemic will not be forgotten and will motivate governments to both take measures to guard against future outbreaks and embrace the guidance of public health professionals.

The following measures can help ensure that the threat of terrorist use of biological weapons remains low. This is by no means an exhaustive list, but it reflects a starting point for emerging policy discussions about how to reduce the chances of a future pandemic and improve capabilities if one occurs. These same measures offer some dual-use benefits to detect terrorist attack with biological agents and improve response capabilities in that unlikely event.

Although these measures are valuable, they cannot override the impact of poor decisions made for political expedience. What is particularly frustrating about the COVID-19 outbreak is that many scholars, public health officials, and intelligence analysts issued repeated warnings about the prospect of a naturally occurring pandemic. With the exception of 2007, every annual statement by the Director of National Intelligence to the U.S. Congress since 2006 has stated that a global pandemic posed a formidable risk to the United States and to the international community. Repeated outbreaks of infectious diseases since 2000 motivated senior planners in the White House to alert senior officials to the prospect of a pandemic. The SARS outbreak in 2002–2003 caused White House officials in the Bush administration to draw up extensive plans to handle a pandemic.[4] Plans were revised early in the Obama administration. Unfortunately, as with other policies and plans from previous administrations, the Trump administration "jettisoned the Obama playbook" on how to manage a pandemic.[5] In April 2018, President Trump's newly appointed national security adviser fired or demoted everyone on the White House's national security team because, as Michael Lewis describes in his history of the U.S. response to the pandemic, "the only serious threats to the American way of life came from other states" and the focus should be "on hostile foreign countries rather than, say, natural disasters or disease."[6] Unfortunately, these warnings and

---

[4] Lewis, 2021, pp. 74–122.

[5] Wright, 2020.

[6] Lewis, 2021, p. 163.

recommendations to prepare for a large-scale outbreak have all too often been overshadowed by calls to prepare for traditional security threats from states or terrorist attacks involving military-grade biological weapons. The shadow of 9/11 and the shock of that attack have had a profound influence on how U.S. leaders and the American public have viewed risk in the past two decades.

Even when recommendations are few and specific, getting them acted on is difficult. Leaders have traditionally paid more attention to the threat of a terrorist attack with a virus or bacteria than to a naturally occurring event. Given this history, care should be taken not to inflate the threat of bioterrorism simply because the globe is bedeviled by a pandemic. In 2005, Leitenberg argued that federal expenditures "to procure vaccines against BW [biological weapon] 'select agents'" would not be nearly as useful as "procuring vaccines against pandemic flu strains" and that U.S. government "reconsideration and redirection should be an urgent executive and legislative priority."[7]

Recommendations

Review and Enhance Controls

Controls on high-containment biological labs, pathogen collections, and laboratory equipment that could be used for pernicious purposes could be reviewed and enhanced to limit danger. There is inherent tension between the desire to avoid hindering legitimate biotechnology and medical research and establishing good security practices. Although the number of high-containment biological lab facilities was increasing significantly before the COVID-19 pandemic, this number is likely to increase even more post-pandemic as countries reevaluate their public health and scientific capabilities to contend with a future outbreak. Many new facilities will be in countries that have not had much experience managing these types of facilities. The possibility of a lab leak or diversion increases as the number of facilities around the globe increases.

---

[7] Leitenberg, 2005, p. 90.

The proliferation of labs will also place greater demands on pathogen collections to supply them. As new facilities with dangerous materials are established, there will be inherent risks of accidents resulting from poor handling procedures relating to the newness of the facility, insider threats, and possible external attack by terrorists or criminals to obtain deadly materials.[8] The 2001 anthrax attacks in the United States is a prime example of the potential danger that might result as the number of facilities increases and facility control and management is not perfect. Moreover, as one researcher noted "there is always the risk that some laboratories will work with pathogens that they are not certified for."[9]

Rules, regulations, and best practices—like all factors that limit risk—can reduce the danger of an inadvertent accident or a determined insider, but they cannot eliminate it. Managing risk calls for enforcing a series of measures that reduces errors and the possibility of intentional pernicious acts. Reviewing and reinforcing the international standards on lab management and pathogen control is essential as the number of these facilities increases around the globe.[10]

Improve Collaboration

Expand collaboration between the animal health and human health sectors. In the past 20 years, multiple outbreaks of zoonotic diseases have occurred. Rift Valley fever, SARS, Middle East respiratory syndrome coronavirus, various types of influenza (H1NI, H5N1, and H7N9), and West Nile virus are all believed to be zoonotic transfers from animals to humans. The origin of COVID-19 is still unclear, but a zoonotic transmission is a

---

[8] Jonathan B. Tucker, "Preventing the Misuse of Pathogens: The Need for Global Biosecurity," *Arms Control Today*, June 2003. Also see John Parachini, "Access and Control of Dangerous Biological Materials in California," in K. Jack Riley and Mark Hanson, eds., "The Implications of the September 11 Terrorist Attacks for California: A Collection of Issue Papers," Santa Monica, Calif.: RAND Corporation, IP-223-SCA, 2002.

[9] Alexandra Peters, "The Global Proliferation of High-Containment Biological Laboratories: Understanding the Phenomenon and Its Implications," *Revue Scientific et Technique*, Vol. 37, No. 3, January 2019, p. 864.

[10] Gregory D. Koblentz and Filippa Lentoz, "Whether Covid Came from a Leak or Not, It's Time to Talk About Lab Safety," *The Guardian*, June 15, 2021.

possibility. If the origin of the disease is the result of a lab leak from a facility in Wuhan, China, the researchers were working on viruses taken from bats in the wild, making it a zoonotic transmission. The possibility does exist that the virus was manipulated as part of a gain-of-function project, which would mean it was not a zoonotic transmission. Regardless of COVID-19's origin, population growth, migration, and climate change are bringing humans in closer contact with wild animals, and this will inevitably lead to higher risks of zoonotic disease outbreaks.

Understanding this risk and being able to identify it early through better disease surveillance capabilities will provide a public health need and serve as a biodefense mission. The One Health Initiative is a worthy effort that seeks to expand "interdisciplinary collaborations and communications in all aspects of health care for humans, animals and the environment."[11] Bringing together a community of interest to connect human and animal health domains is essential as climate change advances and humans push deeper into previously untouched natural areas. Better disease surveillance, containment, and treatment measures also might enhance capabilities to detect suspicious interest in zoonotic diseases and contend with their weaponization in the unlikely event that should occur. Better measures to address natural disease occurrences might also contribute to opposition to the use of exotic diseases and poisons as weapons.

Prioritize Threats

Place higher priority on two near-term threats that the IS and al-Qaeda might inflict on the global community. Near-term threats from the IS and al-Qaeda, such as the use of drone attacks or other strikes on prisons and refugee camps to free their members, warrant more attention than the prospect of the global pandemic stimulating bioterrorism.[12] Since the 2003 U.S. military operations in Iraq, prison breaks have led to repeated resurgences of terrorists and insurgent groups. The number of IS and al-Qaeda members infected with COVID-19 is not publicly known, but the condi-

---

[11] One Health Initiative, homepage, undated.

[12] Bennett Clifford and Caleb Weiss, "'Breaking the Walls' Goes Global: The Evolving Threat of Jihadi Prison Assaults and Riots," *CTC Sentinel*, Vol. 13, No. 2, February 2020.

tions inside the prisons and camps where IS members increase the chances of the virus spreading. Fear of the disease spreading to members detained in these places might have contributed to a sense of urgency to attack. The IS repeatedly urges its followers to free their fellows from captivity. Security at prisons and detention camps with IS and al-Qaeda members should be part of the global counterterrorism plan.

The use of crudely armed drones also poses a near-term threat. Both the IS and al-Qaeda have employed drones in their activities.[13] The IS demonstrated in Iraq and Syria that it could adapt commercially available drones to carry explosives and terrorize and kill people. Drone technology is widely available and the proliferation of more-capable systems that can be modified for weapon delivery is much more likely in the near term than a terrorist attack with a biological agent.[14] Countries with existing controls on commercially available drones should reevaluate their regulatory scheme in light technology and use developments.[15] Better export controls and means of tracking the use of commercially available drones is a necessary step to limit their pernicious use.

Strengthen Norms

Reinforce international norms against state use of chemical and biological weapons. It is essential to reduce interest in the use of biological materials as a means of killing or terrorizing others to redress grievances or pursue religious or political motives—whether it be state actors or nonstate actors (such as insurgent movements). Future meetings and review conferences of the OPCW or of the state parties to the Biological Weapons Convention pose opportunities for states to reinforce the norm. The OPCW, in conjunction with the United Nations, has been investigating the Syrian govern-

---

[13] Abdul Basit, "The COVID-19 Pandemic: An Opportunity for Terrorist Groups?" *Counter Terrorist Trends and Analyses*, Vol. 12, No. 3, April 2020.

[14] Bradley Wilson, Shane Tierney, Brendan Toland, Rachel M. Burns, Colby Peyton Steiner, Christopher Scott Adams, Michael Nixon, Raza Khan, Michelle D. Ziegler, Jan Osburg, and Ike Chang, *Small Unmanned Aerial System Adversary Capabilities*, Santa Monica, Calif.: RAND Corporation, RR-3023-DHS, 2020.

[15] Therese Marie Jones, *International Commercial Drone Regulation and Drone Delivery Services*, Santa Monica, Calif.: RAND Corporation, RR-1718/3-RC, 2017.

ment's gross violations of the Chemical Weapons Convention, and many states have imposed sanctions on the regime. The actions of the OPCW serve to remind the international community that use of these weapons will be investigated and, if found to exist, will lead to adverse consequences. The position is reinforced by the international system of states and civil society organizations any time there is an actual or alleged use of poison or disease as a weapon. The OPCW's recent condemnation of Syria is a worthy measure to help reinforce the norm even if it seems like mild punishment for such heinous actions.[16]

Revisit Threat Assessment

Change the conceptual approach to gauging the threat. No single measure is enough. An interconnected web of measures is needed to reduce the risk of terrorist attacks. The pandemic serves as a stark reminder of the importance of assessing relative risk and probability of threats. Thus, identifying policy measures that mitigate *across the spectrum of threats—both natural and perpetrated by people—*is important to acquire the right tools for action.

---

[16] OPCW, Conference of State Parties, "Decision Addressing the Possession and Use of Chemical Weapons by the Syrian Arab Republic," Twenty-Fifth Session, April 21, 2021.

CHAPTER FIVE

Conclusion

Although there have been remarkable advances in biotechnology, experts who suggest that someone with modest knowledge can access the necessary materials and fashion a biological weapon are cavalierly sweeping aside the difficulties involved. If it is as easy as some suggest, then why are there not more examples of nonstate actors pursuing biological weapons? The prospects of an individual or a group successfully accomplishing all the necessary steps are not zero, but given the difficulty involved in developing such weapons and the fact that conventional weapon alternatives are readily available, nonstate actors have routinely chosen other means of attack. Even such terrorist groups as the IS and al-Qaeda, which have not hesitated to commit terrible acts of violence, have not demonstrated a concerted effort to develop biological weapons, and their chemical weapon activities have thus far been much less deadly than their conventional weapon attacks.

Weaponizing biological materials to cause mass casualties requires considerable engineering sophistication that is difficult even for states. Granted, terrorists might need less much time to obtain or produce and weaponize a biological agent because they might be satisfied with a less effective weapon than a state would call for and might be able to achieve their desired ends with imperfect yet still dangerous results. Still, despite assertions that the biotechnology revolution might make it easier for individuals with some biotechnical training to make biological weapons, the empirical record does not confirm this view.[1] To achieve the desired outcome of mass casualties with biological materials, one must overcome several barriers and success-

---

[1] J. Kenneth Wickiser, Kevin J. O'Donovan, Michael Washington, Stephen Hummel, and F. John Burpo, "Engineered Pathogens and Unnatural Biological Weapons: The Future of Synthetic Biology," *CTC Sentinel*, Vol. 13, No. 8, August 2020.

fully complete several necessary steps. This combination of barriers and steps creates inherent difficulties in the intentional use of biological agents as weapons and makes achievement of desired outcomes uncertain.

Prioritizing threats is a difficult task, particularly when threats are novel. Although individuals and reports issued warnings about the possibility of a pandemic, other near-term or long-feared postulated threats took precedent. Slow-moving and naturally occurring events rarely get the same attention as hostile states or terrorist groups, and feared "bolt from the blue" attacks from states or terrorists dominated the thinking of political leaders and national security experts. COVID-19 and the effects of global climate change are prompts to reimagine threats to national and international security.

When we review both the historical baselines and the pandemic-era narratives of the IS and al-Qaeda, neither group seems likely to use biological materials in future attacks. All the intelligence monitoring and counterterrorism protective measures aligned against them effectively serve to detect a change in their rhetoric or their capabilities. This monitoring, increased public health sensitivity to naturally occurring outbreaks, safeguarding of laboratories researching infectious diseases, and better capabilities to manage the results of an outbreak all combine to lower the risk of the IS, al-Qaeda, or people they might inspire to develop and use biological agents as weapons.

The silver lining of the COVID-19 pandemic is that the international community can rethink the importance of basic public health challenges. States can acknowledge that the low probability of a nonstate actor using biological agents, however frightening, should not overshadow threats of greater probability that now seem all too obvious.

Abbreviations

9/11	September 11, 2001, terrorist attacks
COVID-19	coronavirus disease 2019
IS	Islamic State
OPCW	Organisation for the Prohibition of Chemical Weapons
SARS-CoV-2	severe acute respiratory syndrome coronavirus 2
WMD	weapons of mass destruction

References

Ahmad, Jared, "Serving the Same Interests: The Wood Green Ricin Plot, Media-State-Terror Relations and the 'Terrorism' *Dispotif*," *Media, War & Conflict*, Vol. 12, No. 4, 2019, pp. 411–434.

Al-Qaeda, "The Way Forward: A Word of Advice on the Coronavirus Pandemic," statement, March 31, 2020.

Al-Tamimi, Aymenn Jawad, "Islamic State Advice on Coronavirus Pandemic," blog post, March 12, 2020a. As of December 20, 2020:
http://www.aymennjawad.org/2020/03/
islamic-state-advice-on-coronavirus-pandemic

Al-Tamimi, Aymenn Jawad, "Islamic State Editorial on the Coronavirus Pandemic," blog post, March 19, 2020b. As of December 20, 2020:
http://www.aymennjawad.org/2020/03/
islamic-state-editorial-on-the-coronavirus

Barry, John M., "1918 Revisited: Lessons and Suggestions for Further Inquiry," in Stacey L. Knobler, Alison Mack, Adel Mahmoud, and Stanley M. Lemon, eds., *The Threat of Pandemic Influenza: Are We Ready? Workshop Summary*, Washington, D.C.: National Academies Press, 2005. As of July 29, 2021:
https://www.ncbi.nlm.nih.gov/books/NBK22156/

Basit, Abdul, "The COVID-19 Pandemic: An Opportunity for Terrorist Groups?" *Counter Terrorist Trends and Analyses*, Vol. 12, No. 3, April 2020.

Benjamin, Daniel, "Terrorist Groups: The Quest for Apocalyptic Capabilities," in Kurt M. Campbell, ed., *The Challenge of Proliferation*, Queenstown, Md.: Aspen Strategy Group, 2005.

Binder, Markus K., Jillian M. Quigley, and Herbert F. Tinsley, "Islamic State Chemical Weapons: A Case Contained by Its Context?" *CTC Sentinel*, Vol. 11, No. 3, March 2018.

Binding, Lucia, "Coronavirus: Two Charged with Terror Offenses over Threats to Spread COVID-19, *Sky News*, April 10, 2020.

Bok, Karin, Sandra Sitar, Barney S. Graham, and John R. Mascola, "Accelerated COVID-19 Vaccine Development: Milestones, Lessons, and Prospects," *Immunity*, August 10, 2021.

Carus, W. Seth, "The Rajneeshees (1984)," in Jonathan B. Tucker, ed., *Toxic Terror: Assessing Terrorist Use of Chemical and Biological Weapons*, Cambridge, Mass.: MIT Press, 2000, pp. 115–138.

Carus, W. Seth, *A Short History of Biological Warfare: From Pre-History to the 21st Century*, Washington, D.C.: Center for the Study of Weapons of Mass Destruction, Occasional Paper No. 12, August 2017.

Clapper, James R., "Remarks as Delivered by The Honorable James R. Clapper, Director of National Intelligence, Senate Select Committee on Intelligence— IC's Worldwide Threat Assessment, Opening Statement," Washington, D.C., February 9, 2016, p. 3. As of October 23, 2016:
https://www.dni.gov/files/documents/
2016-02-09SSCI_open_threat_hearing_transcript.pdf

Clifford, Bennett and Caleb Weiss, "'Breaking the Walls' Goes Global: The Evolving Threat of Jihadi Prison Assaults and Riots," *CTC Sentinel*, Vol. 13, No. 2, February 2020.

Commission on the Intelligence Capabilities of the United States Regarding Weapons of Mass Destruction, Report to the President of the United States, March 31, 2005. As of July 21, 2020:
https://www.govinfo.gov/app/details/GPO-WMD

Cruickshank, Paul, and Don Rassler, "A View from the CT Foxhole: A Virtual Roundtable on COVID-19 and Counterterrorism with Audrey Cronin, Lieutenant General (Ret) Michael Nagata, Magnus Ranstorp, Ali Soufran, and Juan Zarate," *CTC Sentinel*, Vol. 13, No. 6, June 2020, p. 8. As of December 20, 2020:
https://ctc.usma.edu/june-2020/

Cullison, Alan, "Inside Al-Qaeda's Hard Drive: Budget Squabbles, Baby Pictures, Office Rivalries—and the Path to 9/11," *The Atlantic*, September 2004. As of August 19, 2021:
https://www.theatlantic.com/magazine/archive/2004/09/
inside-al-qaeda-s-hard-drive/303428/

Danzig, Richard, Marc Sageman, Terrance Leigh, Lloyd Hough, Hidemi Yuki, Rui Kotani and Zachary M. Hosford, *Aum Shinrikyo: Insights into How Terrorists Develop Biological and Chemical Weapons*, 2nd ed., Washington, D.C.: Center for New American Security, December 2012.

Edwards, Jay, and Benoît Gomis, *Islamic Terrorism in the UK Since 9/11: Reassessing the "Soft" Response*, London: Chatham House, International Security Program Paper, ISP PP2011/03, June 2011.

Flade, Florian, "The June 2018 Cologne Ricin Plot: A New Threshold in Jihadi Bio Terror," *CTC Sentinel*, Vol. 11, No. 7, August 2018.

Franz, David R., "Biological Security and Health in the Post-Pandemic World: The Infectious Disease Community's 'Mushroom Cloud'?" *CBW Magazine*, Vol. 13, No. 2, January–June 2020.

Hamby, Chris, and Sheryl Gay Stolberg, "Preparing for Bioterror, Neglecting Virus Threat," *New York Times*, March 7, 2021.

Hanna, Andrew, "Islamists Imprisoned Across the Middle East," Woodrow Wilson Center, June 24, 2021. As of August 19, 2021: https://www.wilsoncenter.org/article/islamists-imprisoned-across-middle-east

Harris, Elisa D., "Threat Reduction and North Korea's CBW Program," *Nonproliferation Review*, Vol. 11, No. 3, Fall/Winter 2004.

Hoffman, Bruce "Why Terrorists Don't Claim Credit," *Terrorism and Political Violence*, Vol. 9, No. 1, Spring 1997, pp. 1–6.

Human Rights Watch, "Thousands of Foreigners Unlawfully Held in NE Syria," March 23, 2021. As of July 22, 2021: https://www.hrw.org/news/2021/03/23/thousands-foreigners-unlawfully-held-ne-syria#

Jenkins, Brian Michael, and Joseph Trella, *Carnage Interrupted: An Analysis of Fifteen Terrorist Plots Against Public Surface Transportation*, San Jose, Calif.: Mineta Transportation Institute, Report 11-20, April 2012.

Jones, Therese Marie, *International Commercial Drone Regulation and Drone Delivery Services*, Santa Monica, Calif.: RAND Corporation, RR-1718/3-RC, 2017. As of October 19, 2021: https://www.rand.org/pubs/research_reports/RR1718z3.html

Jordan, Douglas, Terrence Tumpey, and Barbara Jester, *The Deadliest Flu: The Complete Story of the Discovery and Reconstruction of the 1918 Pandemic Virus*, Washington, D.C.: Centers for Disease Control and Prevention, National Center for Immunization and Respiratory Diseases, December 17, 2019.

Kadlec, Robert, testimony of Dr. Robert Kadlec before the Subcommittee on Emergency Preparedness, Response, and Communications, Committee on Homeland Security, House of Representatives, 113th Congress, 2nd session, Washington, D.C., February 11, 2014.

Karmon, Ely, *The Radical Right's Obsession with Bioterrorism*, Israel: International Institute for Counter-Terrorism, June 2020. As of May 27, 2021: https://www.ict.org.il/Article/2566/The_Radical_Right_and_the_Obsession_with_Bioterrorism#gsc.tab=0

Knights, Michael, and Alex Almeida, "Remaining and Expanding: The Recovery of Islamic State Operations in Iraq in 2019-2020, *CTC Sentinel*, Vol. 13, No. 5, May 2020.

Koblentz, Gregory D., and Stevie Kiesel, "The COVID-19 Pandemic: Catalyst or Complication for Bioterrorism?" *Studies in Conflict & Terrorism*, July 14, 2021. As of July 29, 2021: https://www.tandfonline.com/doi/pdf/10.1080/1057610X.2021.1944023

Koblentz, Gregory D., and Filippa Lentoz, "Whether Covid Came from a Leak or Not, It's Time to Talk About Lab Safety," *The Guardian*, June 15, 2021.

Kruglanski, Arie W., Rohan Gunaratna, Molly Ellenberg, and Anne Speckhard, "Terrorism in Time of the Pandemic: Exploiting Mayhem," *Global Security: Health, Science and Policy*, Vol. 5, No. 1, October 2020.

Lall, Rashmee Roshan, "In Time of Coronavirus, ISIS Shows Method in Its Murderous Madness," *The Arab Weekly*, March 22, 2020. As of December 20, 2020:
https://thearabweekly.com/
time-coronavirus-isis-shows-method-its-murderous-madness

Lee, ArLuther, "Obama Warned of Pandemic Threat in 2014 but Republicans Blocked Funding," *Atlanta Journal-Constitution*, April 15, 2020. As of July 30, 2021:
https://www.ajc.com/news/
obama-warned-pandemic-threat-2014-but-republicans-blocked-funding/
dh2H9HxiuBY05T5uPqtqpI/

Leitenberg, Milton, *Assessing the Biological Weapons and Bioterrorist Threat*, Carlyle, Pa.: Strategic Studies Institute, U.S. Army War College, 2005. As of December 20, 2020:
https://ssi.armywarcollege.edu/
assessing-the-biological-weapons-and-bioterrorism-threat/

Leonhardt, David, "A Complete List of Trump's Attempts to Play Down Coronavirus: He Could Have Taken Action. He Didn't," *New York Times*, March 15, 2020.

Lewis, Michael, *The Premonition: A Pandemic Story*, New York: W.W. Norton & Company, 2021.

Lurie, Nicole, Melanie Saville, Richard Hatchett, and Jane Halton, "Developing Covid-19 Vaccines at Pandemic Speed," *New England Journal of Medicine*, May 21, 2000. As of August 19, 2021:
https://www.nejm.org/doi/pdf/10.1056/NEJMp2005630?articleTools=true

McCarty, Aidan, "Changes in U.S. Biosecurity Following the 2001 Anthrax Attacks," *Journal of Bioterrorism & Biodefense*, Vol. 9, No. 2, June 25, 2018.

Miller, John Dudley, "Postal Anthrax Aftermath: Has Biodefense Spending Made Us Safer?" *Scientific American*, November 1, 2008. As of August 18, 2021:
https://www.scientificamerican.com/article/postal-anthrax-aftermath/#

Moore, Jack, "ISIS' Chemical Weapons Capability Collapses in Syria After Battlefield Losses," *Newsweek*, August 13, 2017. As of May 27, 2021:
http://www.newsweek.com/isis-chemical-weapons-capability-collapses-after-losses-mosul-and-raqqa-624828

National Commission on Terrorist Attacks Upon the United States, *Final Report of the National Commission on Terrorist Attacks Upon the United States*, Washington, D.C., June 17, 2004.

National Intelligence Council, *Mapping the Global Future: Report of the National Intelligence Council's 2020 Project*, Washington, D.C., NIC 2004-13, December 2004.

One Health Initiative, homepage, undated. As of July 29, 2021:
https://onehealthinitiative.com/

OPCW—*See* Organisation for the Prohibition of Chemical Weapons.

Organisation for the Prohibition of Chemical Weapons, Scientific Advisory Board, "Ricin Fact Sheet," Twenty-First Session, SAB-21/WP.5, February 28, 2014. As of July 27, 2021:
https://www.opcw.org/sites/default/files/documents/SAB/en/sab-21-wp05_e_.pdf

Organization for the Prohibition of Chemical Weapons, Conference of State Parties, "Decision Addressing the Possession and Use of Chemical Weapons by the Syrian Arab Republic," Twenty-Fifth Session, April 21, 2021. As of July 20, 2021:
https://www.opcw.org/sites/default/files/documents/2021/04/c25dec09%28e%29.pdf

Parachini, John, "Comparing Motives and Outcomes of Mass Casualty Terrorism Involving Conventional and Unconventional Weapons," *Studies in Conflict & Terrorism*, Vol. 24, No. 5, 2001.

Parachini, John, "Access and Control of Dangerous Biological Materials in California," in K. Jack Riley and Mark Hanson, eds., "The Implications of the September 11 Terrorist Attacks for California: A Collection of Issue Papers," Santa Monica, Calif.: RAND Corporation, IP-223-SCA, 2002. As of October 19, 2021:
https://www.rand.org/pubs/issue_papers/IP223.html

Parachini, John, "Putting WMD Terrorism into Perspective," *Washington Quarterly*, Vol. 26, No. 4, Autumn 2003, pp. 37–50.

Parachini, John, "Aum Shinrikyo," in Brian A. Jackson, John C. Baker, Peter Chalk, Kim Cragin, John Parachini, and Horacio R. Trujillo, *Aptitude for Destruction*, Vol. 2, *Case Studies of Learning in Terrorist Organizations*, Santa Monica, Calif.: RAND Corporation, MG-332-NIJ, 2005. As of October 14, 2021:
https://www.rand.org/pubs/monographs/MG332.html

Parachini, John, and Katsu Furakawa, "Japan and Aum Shinrikyo," in Robert J. Art and Louise Richardson, eds., *Democracy and Counterterrorism: Lessons from the Past*, Washington, D.C.: U.S. Institute of Peace, January 2007.

Peters, Alexandra, "The Global Proliferation of High-Containment Biological Laboratories: Understanding the Phenomenon and Its Implications," *Revue Scientific et Technique*, Vol. 37, No. 3, January 2019.

Pita, Renè, and Rohan Gunaratna, "Revisiting Al-Qa'ida's Anthrax Program," *CTC Sentinel*, Vol. 2, No. 5, May 2009.

Ralph, Elizabeth, "How Covid-19 Could Give Kim Jong Un a Doomsday Weapon," *Politico*, July 28, 2020. As of December 20, 2020:
https://www.politico.com/news/magazine/2020/07/28/
north-korea-coronavirus-vaccine-385096

Rassler, Don, *The Islamic State and Drones: Supply, Scale, and Future Threats*, West Point, N.Y.: Combating Terrorism Center, July 2018.

Schmitt, Eric, "ISIS Prisoners Threaten U.S. Mission in Northeastern Syria, *New York Times*, May 25, 2020.

Shalala, Donna E., "Bioterrorism: How Prepared Are We?" *Emerging Infectious Diseases*, Vol. 5, No. 4, July–August 1999. As of August 18, 2021:
https://wwwnc.cdc.gov/eid/pdfs/vol5no4_pdf-version.pdf

Smith, George, "The American Way of Bioterror—An A–Z of Ricin Crackpots: Homebrew Poison of Choice to the Hard of Thinking," *The Register*, April 22, 2008.

Sonnemaker, Tyler, "Bill Gates Said He Warned Trump About the Dangers of a Pandemic in December 2016 Before He Took Office," *Business Insider*, May 11, 2020. As of July 30, 2021:
https://www.businessinsider.com/
bill-gates-warned-trump-pandemic-danger-before-took-office-2020-5

Strack, Columb, "The Evolution of the Islamic State's Chemical Weapons Effort," *CTC Sentinel*, Vol. 10, No. 9, October 2017.

Török, Thomas J., Robert V. Tauxe, Robert P. Wise, John R. Livengood, Robert Sokolow, Steven Mauvais, Kristin A. Birkness, Michael R. Skeels, John M. Horan, and Laurence R. Foster, "A Large Community Outbreak of Salmonellosis Caused by Intentional Contamination of Restaurant Salad Bars," *Journal of the American Medical Association*, Vol. 278, No. 5, August 6, 1997, pp. 389–395.

Tu, Anthony T., "Aum Shinrikyo's Chemical and Biological Weapons: More Than Sarin," *Forensic Science Review*, Vol. 26, No. 115, 2014.

Tucker, Jonathan B., "Preventing the Misuse of Pathogens: The Need for Global Biosecurity," *Arms Control Today*, June 2003.

"Tunisia Arrests 2 for Trying to Infect Police with Virus," Agence France Presse, April 16, 2020.

United Nations, "UNICEF Urges Repatriation of All Children in Syria's Al-Hol Camp Following Deadly Fire," *UN News*, February 28, 2021. As of July 22, 2021:
https://news.un.org/en/story/2021/02/1085982

United Nations Secretary-General, "Secretary-General's Remarks to the Security Council on the COVID-19 Pandemic," webpage, April 9, 2020. As of December 20, 2020:
https://www.un.org/sg/en/content/sg/statement/2020-04-09/secretary-generals-remarks-the-security-council-the-covid-19-pandemic-delivered

Warrick, Joby, *Red Line: The Unraveling of Syria and America's Race to Destroy the Most Dangerous Arsenal in the World*, New York: Doubleday, 2021.

Warrick, Joby, "ISIS Used Chemical Weapons on Iraqi Prisoners, U.N. Investigators Find," *Washington Post*, May 13, 2021.

Wickiser, J. Kenneth, Kevin J. O'Donovan, Michael Washington, Stephen Hummel, and F. John Burpo, "Engineered Pathogens and Unnatural Biological Weapons: The Future of Synthetic Biology," *CTC Sentinel*, Vol. 13, No. 8, August 2020.

Willis, Henry H., "Guiding Resource Allocations Based on Terrorism Risk," Santa Monica, Calif.: RAND Corporation, WR-371-CTRMP, March 2006. As of October 19, 2021:
https://www.rand.org/pubs/working_papers/WR371.html

Wilson, Bradley, Shane Tierney, Brendan Toland, Rachel M. Burns, Colby Peyton Steiner, Christopher Scott Adams, Michael Nixon, Raza Khan, Michelle D. Ziegler, Jan Osburg, and Ike Chang, *Small Unmanned Aerial System Adversary Capabilities*, Santa Monica, Calif.: RAND Corporation, RR-3023-DHS, 2020. As of October 19, 2021:
https://www.rand.org/pubs/research_reports/RR3023.html

Wright, Austin L., *Why Do Terrorists Claim Credit? Attack-Level and Country-Level Analyses of Factors Influencing Terrorist Credit-Taking Behavior*, Austin, Tex.: University of Texas at Austin, July 16, 2014.

Wright, Lawrence, "The Plague Year: The Mistakes and the Struggles Behind America's Coronavirus Tragedy," *The New Yorker*, December 28, 2020. As of August 18, 2021:
https://www.newyorker.com/magazine/2021/01/04/the-plague-year

Wright, Susan, "Taking Biodefense Too Far," *Bulletin of the Atomic Scientists*, November/December 2004. As of August 21, 2021:
https://journals.sagepub.com/doi/full/10.2968/060006013